KU-593-787

Overcoming Common Problems

Coping with Difficult Families

DR JANE MCGREGOR
and
TIM MCGREGOR

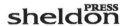
sheldon PRESS

First published in Great Britain in 2014

Sheldon Press
36 Causton Street
London SW1P 4ST
www.sheldonpress.co.uk

Copyright © Dr Jane McGregor and Tim McGregor 2014

All rights reserved. No part of this book may be reproduced or
transmitted in any form or by any means, electronic or mechanical,
including photocopying, recording, or by any information storage and
retrieval system, without permission in writing from the publisher.

The author and publisher have made every effort to ensure that the
external website and email addresses included in this book are correct and
up to date at the time of going to press. The author and publisher are not
responsible for the content, quality or continuing accessibility of the sites.

British Library Cataloguing-in-Publication Data
A catalogue record for this book is available from the British Library

ISBN 978–1–84709–298–4
eBook ISBN 978–1–84709–299–1

Typeset by Fakenham Prepress Solutions, Fakenham, Norfolk NR21 8NN
First printed in Great Britain by Ashford Colour Press
Subsequently digitally reprinted in Great Britain

eBook by Fakenham Prepress Solutions, Fakenham, Norfolk NR21 8NN

Produced on paper from sustainable forests

BURY LIBRARY SERVICE	
Bertrams	10/02/2014
362.82MCG	£8.99

To Fin

Contents

Acknowledgements

We would like to thank our son Fin for his tolerance of us, his sometimes cranky mother and father. No doubt he has material to write an entire book about dealing with difficult parents! We also extend thanks to Fiona Marshall, commissioning editor at Sheldon Press, and Rima Devereaux and Neil Whyte for their invaluable help in editing the book.

1

Introduction

Some family members are difficult to get on with and some are downright antisocial. This is the stuff of family life. It doesn't always have to be harmful. Many of us have family members who push our buttons. It may be the family eccentric – Aunt Martha who lives in a crofter's hut in Scotland without electricity or running water and never exchanges a civil word with the rest of the family; or stingy Uncle Peter, who's so tight he only ever buys the children one small packet of sweets when he arrives for Christmas and always manages to evade paying for anything on family outings; or the family drunk, Grandfather Jo, who given a chance will purloin more than his share of the alcohol at Sunday lunches and launch into a good long natter about himself and his exploits into the bargain. Many families have a professional angry man, like Uncle Martin, alias the Red Mist, who flies into an embarrassing rage if slighted in shops or frustrated by incompetent directions. And many of us have a family bore, whose enthusiasm for pigeon-keeping, golf or whatever is at a rather higher level than the rest of us can maintain.

However, this book isn't really about how to get on with the awkward, opinionated individuals in your everyday home life, who might be irritating but are basically harmless and part of family mythology – though it may well help you have more understanding of them. Families might even be rather dull without their saltier characters, who give the rest of the clan something to gossip about. Such people don't really interfere with your life, or cause you hurt. What we're addressing here are not more or less endearing eccentrics or those with all too human failings whose heart is basically in the right place, but the family member who causes real, long-term distress and affects or restricts your quality of life on a regular, long-term basis: someone who consciously or unconsciously interferes with your freedom and development, and may even appear to be cold, calculating, malicious and cruel; someone who genuinely doesn't seem to have any feeling for others; someone who puts himself or herself first every time and whose big love affair has always been with 'numero uno', and who doesn't seem any too concerned about what happens to the rest of the world. And such people aren't putting it on – they mean it. Hard though it can often be for the rest of us to accept, 'me first' is indeed their motto.

It might be a spouse or partner who routinely belittles you and evades his or her family responsibilities. Or maybe illness, death and inheritance issues have affected your family in a horrible way and the family seems to be falling apart over the issue. Squabbles over wills may be spearheaded by the difficult family member, who always seems to step in and make fresh trouble just when everyone else would be glad to settle things harmoniously. Or perhaps you have demanding, manipulative or even cruel parents or cold siblings, who never really interact with the rest of the family. Or perhaps an elderly parent or parents who have never treated you well are now putting pressure on you to move in because they say they cannot take care of themselves.

What we're talking about are long-term instabilities in your relationship with a family member – someone who's *always* been 'difficult,' no matter how well he or she is treated by life and by others.

George had recently died at the age of 80. His entire family had found him 'difficult' through the generations. From childhood onwards he liked to play the clown for attention, but if this failed there was a notable streak of cruelty and coldness in him. His mother, who said he was always 'peculiar', remembered him as a child deliberately throwing mud over the clean sheets on the line at a time when all the washing had to be done by hand; his younger brother said that the teenage George had once tied him up in the attic and left him there for several hours. In adult life the clowning turned to sarcasm and cutting remarks, often very near the bone, and he seemed to have a knack of insulting people where it most hurt. He did marry happily but his wife found this aspect of him very difficult – the 'little jokes' as she called them – as well as his severely antisocial nature. No one was invited – or allowed – to come to the house. Now it was his children who found this difficult, as well as his moodiness and short fuse. Mealtimes were often a misery and he would easily lose his temper with inanimate objects such as the lawn mower. Needless to say he had quarrelled with his sister and brother and so wasn't on speaking terms with his own family. His peculiarities developed as he grew older, and after his wife died in middle age he cut off all contact with the rest of the family, refusing to see his adult children or to take any interest in his grandchildren. Two years before he died his son made one last attempt and flew over from Canada where he now lived to visit him; George refused to let him in, and died without seeing any of his family again.

Barbara had always found her elder sister Michaela problematic. Although there was only 18 months between them, and they had received exactly the same upbringing, being treated almost like twins, Michaela was from the start marked out by negativity and moodiness. She never quite seemed to find what she was looking for. A successful student, she was invited to apply for Oxbridge but refused, saying she didn't want to be stuck with a load of academic snobs. She worked as a teacher for 20 years and was encouraged to go for a headship, but again refused, on the grounds that she didn't want the responsibility. Her personal life was hard going and lonely. She was engaged to be married for a few months but broke it off, saying he wasn't Mr Right, and thereafter remained single. It was always doubtful whether she would attend family events or whether she would ruin them by arguing with her father, with whom she got on even less well than the rest of the family. At 45 she came into a small legacy and left her job to write textbooks. These were hardly going to be bestsellers, but Michaela now became very cantankerous about her achievements, blaming her parents for everything that had happened – or hadn't happened – in her life. Barbara found this attitude puzzling and unfair – after all, they had had the same parents and upbringing and she, Barbara, was quite different, being busy, outgoing and happy, married with two children and her own design business, which she had used her share of the legacy to start. Barbara increasingly felt that Michaela was on a road to nowhere. Her relations with the rest of the family became very strained, and Barbara was dreading a family week away she had planned to celebrate their parents' wedding anniversary. Michaela was speaking to no one and not returning phone calls or texts. She seemed to have absolutely no consideration for the rest of the family. Frankly, although they were a very close-knit family, Barbara felt it would be a relief all round if she didn't join them.

Laura's mother was a painter. She had had a fair amount of commercial success in her youth but it was never enough. She dramatized herself as an unfairly ignored artist whom no one understood, and the whole world was against. Right from Laura's birth she was incredibly demanding and overprotective of Laura, to the point of abuse – Laura was never allowed to have her bedroom door closed, or to have any real privacy, and had to go to bed early on summer evenings when all the other children were merrily playing in the street. An only child, she was made to feel terribly responsible for her parents' happiness, a dynamic that continued into adult life and became much worse after her father died and she was left with sole emotional responsibility for her mother. Laura didn't want to repeat the pattern of her own childhood, where her own dominating, demanding grandmother had lived with them, but it seemed inevitable and she felt increasingly helpless at her mother's threats to move in with her, her husband and their two children. Emotional blackmail was a routine way of life for Laura's mother, and although Laura knew this intellectually, emotionally she found it almost impossible to stand up to. Laura's mother increasingly blamed her for her own unhappiness and lack of success and fulfilment, and could turn on the tears at the drop of a hat. In vain Laura wore herself to the bone, organizing exhibitions, publicity and web pages for her mother – nothing could make her happy.

Sandra was actively malicious. She schemed to have her brother Dermot put in prison by accusing him of irregularities in the family business. Dermot ran the restaurant ably, if maybe being a trifle sharp about employing immigrant labour, but Sandra would turn up twice or three times a week demanding to see the books and making loud and public scenes, screaming and shouting and even on occasion slapping Dermot. Sure enough they ended up in court, but achieved nothing beyond spending a great deal of money. When Mary, their mother, died, Sandra at once took possession of her flat. There was no will. It was known that Mary kept large amounts of cash in the place but the rest of the family were never to know how much. Sandra used the money to pay for Mary's funeral and other expenses and offered Dermot and their other two siblings an informal and meagre cash settlement on condition that they signed a statement relinquishing all further claim to Mary's estate. Dermot angrily refused and demanded that Mary's affairs be sorted out in a more regular way. That was four years ago, and he has had no contact with Sandra since.

Simon was charming, with a roguish sense of humour and quite a presence, and Sarah Anne was delighted to be married to him. Now her life would blossom as she had always imagined it would, and she eagerly anticipated expanding her career and their joint social life. She was therefore slightly bewildered when somehow this didn't happen. Simon's friends all seemed to melt away after their marriage and Simon kept taking dislikes to her friends and her family, so that they saw increasingly fewer people. In addition Simon would belittle Sarah Anne's work in marketing, calling it trivial and unworthy of her, while her work colleagues were demeaned as 'superficial'. Sarah Anne had been a keen walker but again Simon poured scorn on the group she walked with, calling them a bunch of unfulfilled oddities and eccentrics. Somehow he managed to make himself sound sophisticated and subtle in his criticisms, and apparently quite reasonable, so that Sarah Anne was being increasingly isolated without realizing it. She made new friends with other mothers when their baby was born, but soon gave up her career – without her partner's support it was just too difficult to return to work, and Simon's attitude made it hard for her to see family and friends. After five years of marriage, her life had become smaller rather than bigger.

How do they get away with it, these difficult family members? How do they succeed in establishing such a powerful and dysfunctional dynamic? How do these roles become so entrenched, these tyrannies that, without always being overtly abusive, limit the life and social possibilities of whole families and may be passed down from generation to generation? And more importantly, what can be done about it?

You may be wondering just how possible it is to change what feel like long-entrenched, intractable situations. You may assume it's all your fault and that if you only tried harder all would be well with the difficult family member, or conversely, that you have done your level best and if you could only change the difficult family member, things would be all right. In this book we take a look at common situations where problems are especially likely to arise or worsen if they are not dealt with, and aim to help you address entrenched family issues like those mentioned above.

This book looks at how to survive daily or less frequent interactions with difficult family members. It presents a range of strategies for dealing with family members who push our buttons, and includes real-life advice from people who have successfully overcome family difficulties. Based on the latest research, it looks at a new way of viewing personality types, with a particular focus on the importance of empathy. And if ever you've felt that maybe your difficult family member has a personality problem, you may be right. Several studies over the past decade or so – including ongoing research work by the authors of this book – suggest that difficult family members may often have an undiagnosed personality disorder such as narcissism, or another clinical problem such as Asperger syndrome.

Empathy – the stuff that keeps families together

Empathy is vital for families and society. It acts as social glue and puts the 'kind' in humankind. Without empathy there would be no humanity, just a world of disparate individuals. Imagine what it would be like if we weren't even the slightest bit empathic.

Empathy is the experience of understanding another person's perspective – you place yourself in their shoes and feel what they're feeling. When we empathize we not only mirror the distress of the other person but are moved to respond in socially appropriate ways. In other words, empathy helps us take care of one another. When we are distressed by the suffering of others, that distress becomes the seed of our compassion. Throughout what follows we argue that empathy and compassion are indispensable for strengthening family relations, which is why we place it at the heart of the book.

In all probability empathy developed in the context of parental care. Infants smile and cry in order to urge their parents to help them. The first type of empathy most humans experience is termed **emotional contagion** (the unconscious ability to mimic another person's emotions) and is understood as an innate trait in humans. It is observed, for example, when infants contagiously giggle and gurgle along with other infants. Empathy develops from this early prototype when a child meets normal developmental milestones.

Without the proper mechanism for understanding and responding to our offspring's needs, we humans would not have survived.

Empathy is vital in terms of group (family) survival. One needs to pay close attention to the activities and goals of others to cooperate effectively and thrive as a group. Sometimes our own and others' ability to empathize becomes apparent only when things go wrong, as when we are misjudged by someone else and our feelings get hurt. In these circumstances our response enables the other person to become aware of the misunderstanding and consequences of his or her actions. This ability to share others' feelings betters our understanding of the people around us and promotes cooperative behaviour.

Empathy is fragile though. It is switched on by events within the family or community, such as seeing a child in distress, but it is just as easily switched off if the person in distress happens to be an outsider or someone who has been outcast. Furthermore some people are fantastically empathic when it comes to caring but close down empathy for emotions they are frightened of in themselves, for example if they fear powerful emotions like anger and outrage. So whether you express empathic concern for others in certain situations depends on what you are empathic about and how easy it is for you to feel certain things in your own mind.

Families do not always cooperate – sometimes they compete. In their book *Supercooperators*, Martin Nowak and Roger Highfield state that 'cooperation and competition are forever entwined in a tight embrace'. What they mean is that in pursuing our self-interested goals, we often have an incentive to repay kindness with kindness, so others will do us favours when we are in need.

Competition for survival, by being unhelpful or even attempting to destroy one another, is one of the many thousands of ways that humans compete. We don't just compete by fighting and by being hostile, but also through games, sports, contests and social and career status. And there is good reason for this because being self-interested and low in empathy allows you to act self-interestedly when it is in your best interests to do so, for instance in situations where your life is in danger.

So it's clear there is benefit for both self-interest and empathy in families and everyday life. We can draw on either characteristic at will or as our circumstances dictate. Empathy fosters social cohesion. It means you end up supported by a social network and a family that can be relied on for help so that you don't have to go it alone. Furthermore having a certain amount of empathy means you can avoid offending or inadvertently hurting someone else. Having some amount of self-interest is important too. It ensures that your own needs and wants are not overlooked in favour of the needs of others in the group. It is about finding the right balance. These issues – how to make more of empathy and self-compassion – are discussed in detail in the rest of this book.

2

The empathy spectrum

In this chapter we introduce the idea of an **empathy spectrum** and the personalities dotted along it. We explain the characteristic behaviours of these personalities and provide case studies of some of the more difficult family members you're likely to come across, from the more 'fixed' personalities at the extremes of the spectrum to the more malleable sorts in the middle. We discuss why it isn't just those with too little empathy who are challenging – people with average levels of empathy can prove difficult to deal with as well, as can people at the high end of the spectrum with an abundance of empathy.

Psychology professor Simon Baron-Cohen is best known for studying the theory of 'mind blindness' (a difficulty understanding the thoughts, feelings and intentions of others), which is regarded as key in autistic disorders. In his book *Zero Degrees of Empathy*, Baron-Cohen proposes an empathy circuit in the brain that determines how much empathy we have. He also proposes that there is an empathy spectrum, and each of us is positioned somewhere along it. Imagine this as a gauge with settings on it ranging from zero to six (see Figure 1 overleaf). People who are cruel and lacking in empathy are positioned at one end of the gauge (point zero), whereas people who express empathy in abundance are at the other end (point six). The majority of us are positioned at some point between these two extremes.

We make the empathy spectrum a feature of this book, plotting everyone along it – all the different types of personalities in the family – and using it as a basis to discuss personality traits found from points zero to six. We explore ways of nudging our positions upward, to ease and bring more harmony to strained family relations. And while it's important to improve our compassion and understanding of other people, we also stress the importance of developing more self-compassion to safeguard our own well-being.

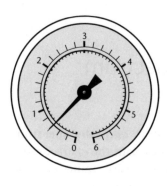

0 No empathy; hurting others means nothing

1 Capable of hurting other people; feels some regret though

2 Enough empathy to refrain from acts of physical aggression

3 Compensates for lack of empathy by covering it up

4 Low to average empathy

5 Slightly higher than average empathy

6 Very focused on feelings of others; almost unstoppable drive to empathize

Figure 1 Points on the empathy spectrum

Points zero to one: The antisocialites

We start at the most challenging end. At **point zero** we have people who have no empathy – apparently none at all. People situated at this point are the sorts who are capable of committing murder. Let's hope there's no one in your family like this! But people with no empathy aren't all murderers. Some are merely incapable of forming relations with other people because they don't understand what the other person is feeling. Many people with no empathy are actually difficult to spot.

We call these people the **antisocialites**. Antisocialites may have diagnosed and undiagnosed personality disorders such as antisocial personality disorder (AsPD). People with antisocial personality disorder are characterized by a long-term pattern of manipulating, exploiting or violating the rights of others. Genetic factors and problems of the social realm such as child abuse are believed to contribute to the development of this condition. Far more men than women are affected, and the condition is common in people caught up in the criminal justice system and those who spend time in prison.

Simon Baron-Cohen defines people with personality disorders like AsPD and psychopathy as **zero negative**. He uses 'negative' because while the individual may enjoy the rollercoaster ride of their own behaviour, it can be an extremely negative experience for those unfortunate enough to be closely involved. Zero-negative conditions also include diagnosable conditions like psychopathy and other disorders of personality including sociopathy, borderline personality disorder and narcissistic personality disorder (see below).

There has been much debate as to the distinctions between this cluster of disorders. For instance, sociopathy is most commonly characterized as a condition where there appears to be something severely wrong with the individual's conscience. Psychopathy is most often characterized as a complete lack of conscience. Clearly there isn't much to separate the two, leaving some people convinced that psychopathy and sociopathy are the same disorder. Alternatively, some regard both as AsPD, while others believe that psychopathic and sociopathic personalities are an extreme version of it, sometimes referred to as dangerous and severe personality disorder (DSPD).

Another condition to add to the antisocialite group is narcissistic personality disorder (NPD), a condition in which people have an inflated sense of self-importance and an extreme preoccupation with themselves. People with NPD tend to react to criticism with rage or humiliation. They often take advantage of other people to achieve their own goals, and have excessive feelings of self-importance. They may have a propensity to exaggerate their achievements and talents. They expect to become a movie star or the next big thing, regardless of whether they have the talent, wealth or wherewithal to go with their dream! In consequence of their grandiosity, they need constant attention and admiration. Narcissistic personality types also often have unreasonable expectations of others, yet paradoxically have a tendency to disregard the feelings of others and exhibit limited empathy largely because of their obsessive self-interest.

Yet another in the mix is people with borderline personality disorder (BPD). Being borderline means individuals often have difficulties controlling their emotions and impulses, and find it hard to sustain relationships. They can experience feelings of emptiness, suffer quick changes in mood and may even harm themselves. It is sometimes called emotionally unstable personality disorder because individuals often experience problems coping with abandonment, and a rapidly changing view of other people can form part of their difficulties.

There is ongoing dispute over the conditions described on the previous pages and whether or not they are distinct disorders. As we have said, they are a confusing mix of terms and sets of behaviours. Nevertheless plenty of people in society have these personality traits, however we choose to define them. Collectively they constitute a larger proportion of the UK general population than might be supposed – in our earlier book, *The Empathy Trap*, we highlighted that up to 4 per cent sit at this end of the spectrum. It is hard to know for sure how many live at large in society because estimates of the extent of the problem are variable, and most if not all the conditions have been subject to redefinition over time. However, we shall attempt to indicate the prevalence of the problem by drawing on the work of academics in this field.

The psychologist Martha Stout, in her book *The Sociopath Next Door*, suggests that as many as 4 per cent of the population come under the antisocial label. This estimate is derived from studies done in the 1990s, most significantly from a large clinical trial carried out by K. L. Barry and colleagues that involved primary-care patients in the USA. It found that 8 per cent of men and 3.1 per cent of women met the criteria for a diagnosis of AsPD. Meanwhile researchers Robert Hare and Paul Babiak estimate that 1 per cent of the population are without conscience, another 10 per cent or more falling into what they call the 'grey zone'. In their book *Snakes in Suits* they suggest that the prevalence is likely to be higher in particular groups and settings such as the business world, where philosophy and practices encourage traits like hardheartedness and greedy behaviour.

It is estimated that 47 per cent of people who meet the criteria for AsPD have significant arrest records. A history of aggression, unemployment and promiscuity is more common than serious crimes among people with AsPD. In the UK the prevalence of AsPD in the general population is 3 per cent in men and 1 per cent in women. If AsPD affects 1 per cent of the general population then that amounts to at least 620,000 people in the UK. So the estimates of antisocial personality disorder and related conditions vary from less than one person in 100 to one person in 25. Worldwide that equates to an estimate of 70 million antisocial individuals.

In Chapter 1 we described George, a quarrelsome and difficult man who died alone at the age of 80 after refusing to let his family see him; Laura's mother, a self-centred and heartless woman; Sandra, who ruthlessly pursued inheritance and then discarded her family when it was clear she wasn't going to get her way; and Simon, who increasingly took control of everything in his wife's life. How are these sorts of personalities to be dealt with? To address this we first need to discuss the types of behaviours and issues that families are commonly confronted with, so next we present three sorts of antisocialite and in each case highlight not only their lack of empathy but specifically the traits that are nearly always present but difficult to spot.

Antisocialite A

Jill is 45, a teacher and a married mother of three teenage boys. It appears no one around her is aware that she is an archetypal sociopath. Outwardly she is respectable, affable and even quite charming. Inwardly she is cold-hearted and behaves unfeelingly whenever she can get away with it. Being devoid of genuine feelings she indeed has a void inside and easily gets bored and listless.

Jill has worked at a local school for two years. It is the longest she has stayed in one job. Despite not enjoying the work or caring for the children in her charge, she persists with it because it provides her with respectability and status. When she can get away with it she will pick on children. The ones she usually targets are the quiet, shy types. She picks on them because she can't stand people who don't have a backbone. Typically she'll do things like downgrade their school work or accuse them of a misdemeanour or for breaking the school rules. She does this just for the sheer pleasure of upsetting them. Her colleagues, even the parents of the children she targets unfairly, are entirely unsuspecting of her true nature because she piles on the charm when it suits. At home her behaviour is not much altered. She doesn't mother her three boys in a 'motherly' or loving way, but is very controlling and manipulative in her dealings with them, especially the eldest because out of the three he is the more quizzical and alert to her games. All three are confused about their feelings for their mother because one minute she showers them with attention and the next she is dismissive and uninterested in them. She relates to her loving husband similarly – grudgingly apprecia-tive of the money and lifestyle his senior executive salary affords while at the same time resenting his lack of verve. Most of the time she feels nothing but contempt for other people.

Commentary

Jill has no conscience about punishing innocent children at school, or about her behaviour to her own children and husband. With little to no empathy for others, even her own family, she uses everyone around her as objects to manipulate. She has no qualms in using her husband to maintain their comfortable lifestyle, experiences no conflict and sees no hypocrisy in presenting the household and everyone in it as the perfect family set-up. She has superficial charm, which she can quickly turn off when someone aggravates her. She seeks out danger and excitement to fill the emotional void, hence her vindictive actions at school. For the time being she mostly limits this side of her character to people and experiences outside the home, but sooner or later her mask will drop and the family may find themselves unprotected and at risk of exposure to the nastier side of her nature. Behind Jill's mask hides an everyday sociopath or psychopath.

Antisocialite B

When we were young, my sister Megan was the one who always got into trouble, both at home and at school – the one everyone talked about. I was embarrassed by her behaviour at times, and we drifted apart because I could no longer cope with her antics – it was emotionally exhausting, the constant up and downs. She was always in some sort of crisis. It wasn't just me, our parents struggled with her and it caused tension at home. Our parents divorced when we were in our teens and since then we've all drifted apart. My brother doesn't have any time for Megan and my father and Megan barely speak. Two of the biggest problems we've had to deal with as a family are the chaos that always surrounds her and her frequent self-harming. It's difficult to comprehend why she does this, and hard to empathize with her over it. She's so changeable and has terrible mood swings. She used to be violent but is less so now. When we were teenagers and living at home I lost count how many times she smashed up her bedroom or cut herself! Nowadays she self-harms less and is less aggressive too, but her chaotic relationships persist. She's in love one minute, on top of the world, letting everyone know how marvellous her new boyfriend is, then before you know it she's slating him and the relationship is over. It's ridiculous – she's so immature, and it's happened so many times! She behaves erratically at work too, and has had so many jobs I've lost count. She's such a pain – I wonder why I bother with her sometimes.

Commentary

Megan has what some doctors call borderline personality disorder, or BPD, and others 'emotionally unstable'. There is an ongoing debate about the terminology of the disorder, especially the word 'borderline'. Symptoms are usually only diagnosed in adults but children and adolescents may exhibit them. People with BPD swing from having positive regard for themselves one minute to self-loathing the next. They feel emotions intensely and their sudden change and lowering of mood can induce self-harming and suicidal behaviour. This may require them to be admitted intermittently to hospital for psychiatric care. How does this affect their ability to empathize with other people? Individuals with BPD can be very sensitive to the way others treat them, but their feelings about others often shift from positive to negative if they perceive that there is a threat of losing someone, or that the person no longer holds them in high regard. Their thinking tends to be black and white and undermines their ability to maintain relationships. All this changeability causes problems for Megan and those around her, as her sister points out.

Antisocialite C

Bob is a divorcee. His only daughter, Amy, fast approaching her tenth birthday, lives with her mother, a placid woman who initially found it hard to disengage from Bob and their marriage but now, after years of pandering to Bob's ego and many whims is enjoying her newfound independence. In general she finds Bob very manipulative so limits their exchanges to conversation about the shared care and the well-being of their daughter. We call Bob a narcissist.

Bob's relationship with his daughter Amy is a complex and confusing one, and she's often left upset by his actions and behaviour. For example, for her birthday and without her knowledge, Bob had Amy's bedroom redecorated in his large and fancy new house (a place he'd recently bought with his latest girlfriend, the fourth partner he'd had since his divorce 18 months ago). By Bob's reckoning the bedroom and its décor was perfect for his little princess. He'd installed an over-the-top fairytale four-poster bed and other expensive furniture. He'd really gone to town and was dying to show it off to her when she came for her weekend stay.

Amy couldn't help but show her surprise and disappointment. She was the least 'girly' girl you could imagine and didn't like it – it was all so over the top: pink walls, a great deal too 'fluffy' and ridiculously extravagant. It didn't feel like her room at all. She was offended by his off-the-cuff remark that he had thrown away her favourite bear, the one she'd had for as long as she could remember. He told her she was too old for that babyish nonsense. She tried to hide her disappointment and longing for familiar things and thanked her father. But all he saw was that she was thoroughly ungrateful, so he raged at his daughter for being selfish.

Commentary

Bob was motivated to decorate Amy's room less by a desire to make his daughter happy and more to show her mother in a bad light – trying to make her look ungenerous and stingy – and perhaps to show his new girlfriend what a great and kindly father he was. Bob is a narcissist. Narcissistic personality disorder (NPD) is a disorder in which individuals are excessively preoccupied with themselves. Historically people with NPD were called megalomaniacs and severely egocentric. Such people have such an elevated sense of self-worth that they overvalue themselves and see themselves as better than others. Yet they can also be fragile and unable to handle criticism, and often compensate for this by belittling others in order to validate their own self-worth. It is this sadistic tendency that is characteristic of narcissists, and hinders them from empathizing with other people. Bob has these traits and while he mostly keeps them under wraps with his new girlfriend, at least in the short term, his less appealing nature and violent rage is revealed in his relations with his daughter and ex-wife.

Points two to three: People with low empathy

Do you have a sibling like Michaela, whom we met in Chapter 1, who is moody, blames others and is more than a little dispirited about life? Or do you have a father, spouse or brother who seems self-absorbed, obsessive? In addition, do they have trouble communicating or showing concern or affection for others? Are they rather cold or aloof, detached from others? We place people with these traits at **points two to three** on the empathy spectrum. In this section and later in Chapters 5 and 6 we consider a range of behaviours that suggest you may be dealing with someone with low empathy. These include behaviours that form diagnosable conditions along the autistic spectrum, such as **Asperger syndrome** (AS), but also individuals who have never been diagnosed with a particular disorder or are even aware that a diagnosable condition could be ascribed to them and their particular behaviours. We also include in our discussion those who experience, temporarily or otherwise, low empathy and those with addiction problems, eating disorders and obsessive–compulsive patterns of behaviour.

Most people with low empathy do have some propensity to empathize, even if this is a response to reasoning as opposed to feelings of concern for another. So we hold the view that people with low empathy are not in an immutable position and can make some real changes to the amount of empathy they express. Likewise we believe that understanding how they view the world will help you empathize with them.

Asperger revisited and the autistic spectrum

In recent years the idea that people with high functioning autism or Asperger syndrome have greatly reduced empathy has been contested. In 2007 the *Journal of Autism and Developmental Disorders* reported a study by Kimberley Rogers and colleagues that showed that while individuals with AS scored lower on some measures of empathy (perspective-taking and the ability to attribute mental states such as beliefs, intents, desires, pretending and knowledge to oneself and others), they were no different from anyone else in their tendency to show empathic concern or personal distress on seeing another person in distress. This and subsequent studies have cast serious doubt on the more traditional view of people with AS having very limited empathy.

Individuals on the autistic spectrum often experience low levels of empathy because their particular style of thinking (cognition), which tends towards excessive attention to details and patterns or rules (Baron-Cohen calls this 'systemizing'), can leave them frustrated and alienated. To understand this we need to think about the autistic spectrum as involving a strong drive to systemize. Though this can have positive consequences for individuals and for society (they might positively contribute to systems of production in the world of work, for example), there is also a downside. People and emotions are hard to systemize! Attempting to systematize others is likely to lead to frustration, and frustration can lead to reduced empathy.

Recent studies also point to some people with conditions like AS being highly empathic. Indeed, some individuals can be oversensitive to the emotions of others and become very upset to learn they have hurt another person's feelings. They may have strong moral consciences and codes and care about not hurting people. They may not always be aware that they have said something rude or hurtful, but if it is pointed out, they would most likely want to do something about it.

Typically, many on the autistic spectrum are not very good at the 'mind-reading' part of empathy. They find it hard to predict people's behaviour and feelings, which is in stark contrast to sociopaths, psychopaths and other antisocialites, who are often expert 'mind readers' but paradoxically show an inability or unwillingness to care. This is why they are good at deception – you have to be good at mind reading before it would even occur to you to deceive some other person. In other words, the perceptive part of empathy seems to function very well in sociopaths/psychopaths, but they don't have the appropriate emotional response to someone else's state of mind – they don't *feel* a need or desire to alleviate distress even if they see someone is in pain. This isn't the case with regard to people with autism or AS or some other state of low empathy. They are more likely to have problems fathoming out whether someone else is in emotional distress (poor mind-reading skills), but once they do comprehend it, they tend to want to alleviate it.

Disorders that sit along the autistic spectrum are regarded by the medical establishment as lifelong developmental ones that affect how individuals communicate with and relate to other people. They also affect how they make sense of the world around them. But because autism is a spectrum condition, while all people with autism share certain difficulties, their condition will affect them in different ways. Some people with autism are able to live relatively independent lives but others may have accompanying learning disabilities and need special support. The family of autistic spectrum disorders known as ASD includes AS. Asperger syndrome is distinguished from autism by the absence of significant language delay, and general intellectual skills tend to be in the normal range. The

National Autistic Society estimates a prevalence rate of people with autistic spectrum disorders of 1 in 100 people.

John is 43, married, and though he doesn't know it, has Asperger syndrome. His wife, Anne, though she finds some of his behaviour somewhat irritating, has never thought of him as personality disordered either. They met when they were in their twenties. He was attentive and loving at first and continued to be during the early years of their marriage. Though socially awkward, he was considerate and kind whenever they were alone together, and Anne, who was not very confident herself but quite stubborn, liked his independent, quirky streak.

A few years down the line Anne found herself often irritated by John's constant grumpiness. She tried to not let it bother her too much and viewed it as something normal to contend with in marriage. However, she was also irritated by John's often obsessive idiosyncrasies. For instance, he was fastidious about lots of things but probably fussiest about what he ate. He obsessed over where they bought their food, the menus, what time they ate, about odours, and was hypervigilant about hygiene in the kitchen. This fastidiousness extended to other things too. He had a tendency to label things, arrange things in order – 'correctly', he would say – and got very stressed if any routine at home was changed. He'd become upset if someone else cooked for him so in general Anne let him cook their meals. It was embarrassing if they went to dinner with friends, as he generally complained or made a fuss.

John also developed a number of compulsive daily rituals. He found it hard to relax and unwind, so he had a set bedtime routine without which he couldn't sleep. Socially he was quite awkward and had no talent whatsoever for small talk. One thing that Anne noticed was that he never looked other people in the eye when he spoke, and often interrupted other people in mid-flow. Another issue of communication was that John took other people's words too literally – he had no idea how to deal with sarcasm or have friendly banter. Generally speaking he was uncomfortable around other people, and that in consequence made others uncomfortable around him. Social situations therefore were a source of stress for him and embarrassment for Anne.

Commentary

It is likely that like John, many adults with AS go undiagnosed throughout their lives. This may or may not be a good thing, depending on your view. They may have impairments in social interaction, including problems maintaining friendships or engaging in activities with others. There are also impairments in communication, as in John's case, where the individual takes whatever is said literally and is unable to read between the lines. This can lead to frustration and affects not just the individual but those with whom he or she comes into contact. In the USA the label AS has been dropped from the latest version of the American Psychiatric Association's Diagnostic and Statistical Manual of Mental Disorders (DSM-V) and replaced with the single diagnostic label of autistic spectrum disorder (ASD). This doesn't automatically affect diagnosis in the UK, where the World Health Organization's International Classification of Diseases (ICD) holds more sway. The ICD description is also slightly different anyway. Furthermore any changes to the WHO's classification will not occur until 2015. The autistic spectrum and AS are discussed again in Chapter 5.

Points four to low-five: The in-betweeners

At **points four to five** on the empathy spectrum are the group of people we term the in-betweeners – people of average or normal levels of empathy. This might seem a good and safe place to be positioned as far as the issue of empathy goes, and in many respects that perception would be quite right. But even here at this middling position, people can experience problems expressing empathy.

> Andy is a single parent and regards himself as a good father to Marie, his 15-year-old daughter and only child. However, recently he has noticed she is starting to look very thin but he doesn't want to ask her about her dieting. In truth he is more than a little afraid to ask as she has seemed a bit distant and grumpy over the past three months. Nevertheless he persuades himself that it will pass and is most likely just normal adolescent behaviour.
>
> One day recently Marie's best friend Jane stayed for a sleepover. After they had eaten, Andy overheard Jane telling Marie that she needed to get help for her eating disorder, and advised her to discuss it with her dad or the family doctor. Marie refused and said that her dad didn't either know or really care about her, or whether she was eating properly.
>
> But even after overhearing this, Andy does nothing. He doesn't want to have an argument with his daughter as still views her as 'his little girl'. This stops him from acknowledging that she is obviously unhappy and harming herself by not eating.

Over the next two months Marie continues to lose more weight and is beginning to look startlingly thin. Andy doesn't want to rock the boat and so still doesn't confront the situation.

Commentary

Many of us would find it difficult to deal with a situation like Andy's, and like him might opt to keep quiet about being aware of the problem his daughter Marie is facing. Nevertheless his inaction amounts to apathy.

Let's look closer at apathy and its consequences in everyday situations. The word apathy is derived from the Latin *apathīa* and Greek *apátheia*, meaning an insensibility or indifference to suffering. In the context of everyday life it means we lack interest in or concern for things that others are moved or excited by. Some view apathy as akin to stoicism, meaning being free from emotion of any kind; however, most view it as a temporary affliction, say as a first reaction to danger.

Apathy can be an avoidance strategy, engaged in in the hope that the problem will go away. Apathetic people are often fearful people – individuals who don't perceive of themselves as having the necessary resources to confront a difficult situation or challenge. The avoidance strategy is often favoured because a danger is no longer important if its existence is denied. Andy avoids being drawn into an awkward situation and danger by surrendering to a state of 'learned helplessness'. He keeps quiet out of fear, perhaps, that confronting the issue with Marie would harm their relationship. He may also be fearful of facing the fact that his daughter could be seriously damaging her well-being and health.

Apathy is also a common trait of 'people pleasers' – individuals who act in flattering and ingratiating ways to avoid conflict with other people. Apathy is the number one foe of those seeking to build a more empathic society. Its prevalence is one of the main reasons bullies and abusers get away with mistreating others. If most of us were in a permanent state of trepidation and responded like this, with apathy, tyranny would rule the world.

In *The Empathy Trap* we introduced the word 'apath' to our vernacular as a noun to denote those who turn a blind eye to abuse. We used it then and apply it now to people who are usually empathic, just not in particular circumstances. To highlight the problem of apathy we used the analogy of the tale 'The Emperor's New Clothes' by Hans Christian Andersen. In the tale two weavers promise the Emperor a new suit of clothes that is invisible to people who are stupid. When the Emperor parades before his subjects all the adults, not wishing to be seen in a negative light, pretend they see the Emperor's elegant new clothes. From infancy we are trained to conform to society's standards and rules and conditioned to keep quiet, which often means turning a blind eye or putting up with abuse. In other words, we are moulded into apaths – the folk who pretend not to see that the Emperor is naked. In Chapters 7 and 8 we examine apathy in more detail and suggest ways that people like Andy can learn to put apathy aside when empathy and action are needed.

Points high-five to six: empaths and superempaths

At higher-than-average **point five** we have **empaths** and higher still, at **point six** (and somewhat arbitrarily because the threshold between 5 and 6 is blurry), we have **superempaths**, people who are exceptionally empathic. In our context empaths are ordinary people who are perceptive and insightful, who frequently respond to their gut reactions or instincts. Going back to 'The Emperor's New Clothes', an empath is the boy who utters the unmentionable – that the Emperor isn't wearing any clothes. Empaths combine the attributes of **emotional intelligence** and empathy. This affords empaths the ability to understand their own emotions, listen and empathize with other people, express their emotions productively and in so doing, improve their personal power and their relations with other people.

While words may mask many people's true emotions, empaths intuitively pick up the true notes of emotions behind the words. To put it another way, they are perceptive. The highly sensitive person – a term used interchangeably with empath – is thought to make up 15 to 20 per cent of the population. According to the psychologist Elaine Aron of York University in Toronto, people are born this way. She points out that biologists have found similar behaviour in a multitude of animals, from fruit flies to primates. The trait may reflect a certain type of survival strategy, that of being observant before acting (Aron 1996).

Some empaths feel things particularly strongly, and can pick up other people's inner turmoil. This type of personality is sometimes referred to as a superempath, and such people are positioned at the extreme high end of the spectrum at point six. Super vigilant types like these are more aware than most of subtleties, tend to reflect on things more deeply, and are easily overwhelmed – if you notice everything, you are naturally going to be overstimulated.

Superempaths are not a new species, though they have been sorely misunderstood in the past. They are often typecast as extremely and overly sensitive, prone to shyness and introversion (timidity), though in fact 30 per cent of superempaths are extrovert (outgoing). Having said that, sensitivity is indeed a defining feature of the superempath, and is valued differently in different cultures. In cultures where sensitivity is not valued, superempaths tend to have low self-esteem. They are told 'Don't be so sensitive', so many are left feeling abnormal and can become demoralized if misjudged in this way.

And this is why **point six** on the empathy spectrum is placed not far from **point zero** on the empathy gauge – in fact on our gauge (see Figure 1) they are practically next to one another. In extreme circumstances and under duress, individuals with high empathy may develop considerable social anxiety, to the point that it turns into social phobia and a desire to retreat into themselves. Under these conditions superempaths may shun other people and appear to behave in as self-absorbed and wounded way as, say, a narcissist with crushed self-esteem and zero or very limited empathy!

Yet despite the misunderstandings, high empathy is anything but a flaw. Many individuals who see life through empathic eyes are unusually creative and gifted on account of their emotional intelligence. They often make good peacemakers. Superempaths include South African Archbishop Desmond Tutu and the Dalai Lama. Nonetheless, few superempaths profit so well from their talents. Without proper understanding of their own gifts, many experience frustration and misunderstanding. We consider their particular problems in Chapters 9 and 10, where we offer strategies to help them make the most of their special insight.

Barry is a kindly man in his eighties with two grown-up daughters and eight grandchildren. He has recently lost the love of his life, Eileen, his wife of 50 years.

His loss feels unbearable. Eileen was the only one who truly understood Barry's generous yet super-sensitive nature. She would protect him from the world if he got overwhelmed in caring and looking out for others. Barry is best described as a 'salt of the earth' character – the sort to put others' needs before his own. The only person who Barry let care for him was Eileen, and now he is on his own.

Barry didn't like people fussing around him or being the centre of attention. He preferred to spend a lot of time each day on his own in the garden shed. Eileen had instinctively known he needed time to recharge his emotional batteries. But after her death no one was there to look out for Barry and help prevent him overdoing things, so it wasn't long before he felt emotionally spent, missing the restorative power of time out. His daughters suggested he stay with them for a while but he refused. Two weeks later his eldest daughter went to see him after he didn't answer her phone calls, and found him barricaded in the garden shed. It was clear that he had been drinking heavily and was in a state of extreme distress. It was some time before she managed to get him to come out, and it took more time still before he began to cope better with his grief and depression. It was difficult for all the family to cope with the changes in their father/grandfather while they also were coming to terms with their own loss and grief.

Commentary

Barry is a typical empath. He finds it hard to put his needs first and think about himself. For years he compensated for this lack of self-compassion by having a supportive and compassionate wife. Alone suddenly after Eileen's death he has fewer means of moderating his emotions, which suddenly and overwhelmingly go into overdrive as he goes through the process of grieving. His response is to escape to the garden shed and avoid other people. Increasingly isolated, he is cut off from support and becomes depressed. Barry needs to start practising more self-compassion if he is to grieve properly and come to terms with the loss of his wife. His drinking, erratic moods, reclusive and inward-looking behaviour are all new challenges for the family to contend with.

3

The antisocialites

This chapter focuses on the ups and downs of living with anti-socialites, the group with antisocial traits on points zero to one on the empathy spectrum like those mentioned in Chapter 1 – Laura's mother who treated her daughter coldly; Sandra who fought her family over their mother's will; Simon with a tendency to belittle his wife. These types were also highlighted by way of three more case studies in Chapter 2 – Jill the cold mother and sociopath who enjoys playing cruel games on the children at school; Megan who self-harms and has mood swings; Bob the self-absorbed parent. Some people in this group have diagnosable conditions – socio-paths, narcissistic personalities – while others have antisocial personality traits that persist despite a lack of diagnosis or close fit with a medically defined disorder. What they all have in common is that none show any or very little empathy or regret about the effect of their actions on other people.

You may assume the problems you face with your family member are your fault and that if you only tried harder or offered one more chance, all would be well and the difficult family member would grant the long withheld love and approval. Or conversely you may feel that you have done your level best and that if you could only change your spouse's or other family mem-ber's behaviour, all would be well. But this is a dangerous view to take, as antisocialites often present a danger to themselves and/or others, so it is important to get to grips with their behaviour traits and put boundaries in place to cope with them. People with no or extremely low levels of empathy are the most worrying of all personalities because relations with them expose you to danger and the risk of abuse. What compounds the problem of living with antisocialites is that they are virtually immune to change – they leave that to the rest of us. It is therefore usually very necessary to instigate boundaries of communication and interaction, if balance and harmony are ever to be established in family life. In this chapter we discuss how easy it is to have your life upturned by an antisocialite, and in the next highlight ways to instil boundaries for the sake of self-preservation.

Sociopathic behaviour

In the case study of Jill in Chapter 2, we referred to her as an archetypal sociopath (see p. 13), yet in her daily life Jill's unseemly behaviour pretty much goes undetected and unchallenged, even by her husband and children. Jill is a teacher at a local school. We describe her outward persona as affable and quite charming. Inwardly, however, she hides an ugly truth; she's cold and remorseless – the hallmarks of the sociopath or psychopath.

In his 1941 book *The Mask of Sanity*, the American psychiatrist Hervey Cleckley first described the diagnostic criteria for the 'psychopathic personality', based on observations of adult male psychopaths hospitalized in a closed institution. Cleckley drew up a set of diagnostic criteria, including superficial charm, a lack of anxiety or guilt, undependability or dishonesty, egocentricity, an inability to form lasting intimate relationships, a failure to learn from punishment, poverty of emotions, a lack of insight into the impact of their behaviour and a failure to plan ahead. Cleckley's definition made no reference to physical aggression or breaking the law, behaviours many people associate with the condition. In a later edition of his book Cleckley described the psychopath as 'a biologic organism outwardly intact, showing excellent peripheral function, but centrally deficient or disabled'. This perfectly describes the personality of our sociopath, Jill, who succeeds in playing the role of perfect wife, mother and teacher well enough to convince most people around her, even though behind the façade lurks a cruel and callous woman.

Sociopathy and psychopathy are often used interchangeably. In fact sociopath and psychopath were both incorporated in the American Psychiatric Association's Diagnostic and Statistical Manual of Mental Disorders definition for antisocial personality disorder (AsPD). Though the diagnostic criteria for AsPD were based in part on Hervey Cleckley's pioneering work on psychopathy, AsPD is not synonymous with psychopathy and the diagnostic criteria are different.

To further muddy the waters, the Association brought out the fifth edition of the Manual, DSM-V, in May 2013. This brings with it major changes to the assessment and diagnosis of personality disorders, too complex to expand on here but which include a revamped diagnostic process involving a dimensional rather than a categorical approach based on the severity of dysfunctional personality trait in various domains. Patients will be assessed on how much they match the prototype personality disorder types (for example, antisocial/psychopathic; borderline; narcissistic).

Many countries outside the USA use the WHO's classification system. Its International Classification of Diseases, tenth edition (ICD-10), defines a disorder similar to antisocial personality disorder called **dissocial personality disorder**, which is characterized by callous unconcern for the feelings of others, a gross and persistent attitude of irresponsibility and disregard for social norms, rules and obligations and such like, amounting to what may be referred to as amoral, antisocial, psychopathic or sociopathic personality disorder.

Probably, then, given the mounting confusion over the terms mentioned here, the best approach is to remove ourselves from the present debate. We shall, however, use the term sociopath for ease of reference for the remainder of the book because we view this kind of personality as lurking within the social body and having relentless interaction with it. In the longer term though, we hope doctors will cease using these confusing terms. Though a formal diagnosis may add credence in court if an individual has committed a crime, it is of little consequence for those who share their lives with personalities like this because not only are there currently no treatments to moderate the worst excesses of these antisocial traits, but antisocialites like this usually don't feel remorse for their actions and are also insensitive to punishment.

And here lies the crux of the problem for the rest of us in society. An antisocialite like Jill may already have inflicted physical and psychological harm on others many times over and long before it comes to the attention of authorities. This means the rest of us need much more of a handle on the traits and patterns of behaviour of antisocialites in order to protect and equip ourselves better for dealing with such people in our lives.

Empathy erosion

In his book *Zero Degrees of Empathy*, which we noted in Chapter 2, Simon Baron-Cohen discusses the notion of empathy erosion, which he says arises when we have corrosive emotions like bitterness or a desire for revenge. In many cases empathy erosion is a temporary affliction – a suggestion we raise in Chapter 7 when we discuss the problem of apathy in people with otherwise decent levels of empathy. But what if empathy erodes because of more permanent psychological characteristics?

According to Baron-Cohen there are ten regions of the brain that make up what he terms the **empathy circuit**. Many of these regions are involved in actively coding our experiences and are automatically active when we perceive others behaving in similar ways or having similar experiences. Neuroimaging (brain-scan) studies lend support to the idea that sociopaths and psychopaths have abnormalities in the empathy circuitry of the brain. It is thought that differences in their brain circuitry account for their lack of reaction to other people's distress. But while scientists have made progress in revealing mechanisms thought to enable a person to feel what another is feeling, the evidence, and our understanding of what helps and hinders empathy, is far from complete. We do not yet have a nuanced understanding of the environmental and biological influences or how they interact.

Can sociopaths and psychopaths turn empathy on and off?

The generally held view is that empathy is a highly flexible phenomenon. Among other things it can be affected by the context of the situation, the relationship between empathizer and the other person and so on. This view is held except in relation to situations where the individual is thought to lack empathy entirely – in other words, those at the extreme end of the spectrum (point zero). In such cases the traditional orthodoxy has it that antisocial personalities like sociopaths and psychopaths are permanently unable to empathize. But a recent study challenges this viewpoint. In fact it arguably demonstrates the reverse – that even sociopaths and psychopaths don't lack empathy and can turn it on when they want to. In 2012 the research neuroscientist Christian Keysers and colleagues from the Netherlands carried out a study that suggests that psychopaths can activate empathy on demand. The study measured the psychopath's empathy for others. The subjects were then told that the study was designed to measure empathy, after which a surprising thing happened: their empathy 'normalized'. The research therefore suggests that psychopaths – sociopaths, our term of choice, in all but name – don't lack empathy, but abnormally suppress it. The suppression mechanism that helps regulate the response in normal people is 'over active' in the case of the sociopath, or so Keyser's findings suggest. When told that they were being studied for empathy, the study participants were apparently able to turn it back on somehow. Some experts have suggested that if this proves true, it raises questions of moral accountability. If certain individuals have a brain chemistry that makes them indifferent to empathic responses and yet they can overcome a lack of empathy when prompted, then the question becomes whether these people are aware of this, and exactly what the mechanism is that turns empathy back on.

Another question this situation triggers is whether, if sociopaths' deficiencies are reduced to defective brain circuitry, the rest of us should be too hasty in castigating them. Wouldn't it be better to seek effective treatments to help them, perhaps focusing on reward-based treatments as opposed to punishment? This may seem a ludicrous and unethical suggestion to propose, given the dangers extreme antisocial types pose, yet is it outside the realm of possibility to imagine movement in levels of empathy for those at point zero? Currently there are no known treatments that produce tangible differences in behaviour or levels of empathy in these personality types, so for now the advice is to view the sociopathic encounter dispassionately and, whenever contact is necessary, establish firm boundaries of interaction and communication.

The sociopathic transaction

In *The Empathy Trap* we focused on the nature of sociopathic abuse – psychological manipulation, emotional and or physical abuse – and how it manifests in everyday life. Here we briefly recapitulate the processes by which sociopaths and quite plausibly other antisocialites go about abusing other people.

Often perceptive and emotionally tuned-in people, which we term **empaths**, are targeted by sociopaths because they pose a significant threat. Empaths may not know it, but their powers of detection and perceptiveness to danger mean they're often the first to detect and act upon a sense that something's not right – they react to their gut instinct. Their forthright actions make them the number-one foe of the sociopath because they are likely to point out situations of danger and ruin the sociopath's sport. Yet empaths are also attractive to sociopaths, for their positive attributes and ethical behaviour may entertain these otherwise bored and listless individuals.

Problems really start for empaths when sociopaths involve other people, often placid and apathetic types. Apathetic people, whom we term apaths, are readily duped by sociopaths and blindly follow their lead. How apaths and otherwise fair-minded people become involved in sociopaths' foul play is not difficult to understand. What renders them willing accomplices to sociopaths is poor judgement resulting from lack of insight. This may be because they feel reduced empathy for the person who is the sociopath's target. They themselves might bear a grudge, be jealous, angry or have a sense of being let down by the targeted person and consequently be as keen as the sociopath to see the individual defeated. At other times it could be because they don't *want* to see 'bad' in others so they choose *not* to see it. It could be that they choose not to see because they have too many issues themselves or because they don't possess the ability or moral courage to help that other person. Whatever the reason for their involvement with sociopaths, what happens is that apaths' consciences fall asleep (we discuss apaths' personalities and apathy in relationships and society in more detail in Chapters 7 and 8).

Apaths, whether unwittingly or not, can become involved in sociopathic abuse of others. This happens when they become part of a toxic situation and threesome we call the **sociopath–empath–apath triad**, or **SEAT**. The usual SEAT set-up goes something like this: an empath, who sees the situation for what it is, makes a stand on seeing the sociopath say or do something untoward or on perceiving a threatening situation – the empath challenges the sociopath. The sociopath shifts the blame or focus on to the empath. The apath corroborates the sociopath's false perspective and the empath is subjected to abuse. Ultimately the situation ends badly for the empath, and sometimes too for the

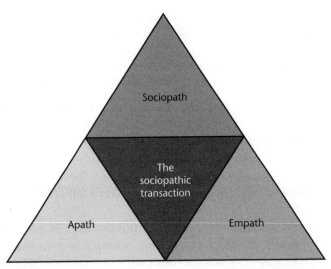

Figure 2 The sociopath–empath–apath triad and sociopathic transaction

apath (particularly if he or she later feels guilty or becomes a target), but frustratingly, the sociopath usually gets off scot-free. This tried and tested formula guarantees the sociopath success. We term the sociopath's manoeuvrings the **sociopathic transaction**. Figure 2 is an illustrative diagram of SEAT and the sociopathic transaction. The apath essentially enters into a pact with the sociopath.

A typical day in the life of Jill, our example of a sociopath from Chapter 2, illustrates how the sociopathic transaction works.

The sociopathic transaction in action

One morning at school a colleague of Jill's turned into the corridor just at the moment Jill began a nasty verbal assault on a child. The teacher knew the child generally to be well behaved, even a little timid, and he couldn't imagine what the little girl could have done to deserve such a dressing down. He was shocked by what he heard and saw.

Jill made excuses about why she was behaving in this extreme way, but her colleague didn't believe her story (she said her actions were justifiable owing to the child's extreme misconduct in class). He ensured that the child was OK, walked her out into the playground to find her friends and told her he would come back to find her once he had discussed the matter with her teacher (Jill). Jill's version of events had left him unconvinced so he sought out the class teaching assistant before attempting to talk to her again. But unbeknown to him Jill had already 'worked' on the teaching assistant, who was new to the post and intimidated enough to go along with Jill's new version of events. So by the time the colleague asked the teaching assistant about what had happened earlier in class, the assistant substantiated Jill's story.

In this situation the **apath** is the teaching assistant who added credence to **sociopath** Jill's story, and the **empath** is Jill's teacher colleague who goes with his gut instinct. Collectively they make up the SEAT. The classroom assistant goes along with Jill's story because unbeknown to the other teacher, she's been on the receiving end of Jill's bullying ways for a while, but is afraid to tell anyone for fear of risking her job.

One of the concerning things about this situation is that without evidence that bullying by the teacher occurred it is unlikely that the situation would be suitably dealt with. It is not uncommon for children to keep quiet about abuse for fear of punishment and not being believed. The little girl is far more likely to internalize her feelings about the incident and feel ashamed.

What research there is on antisocial behaviour like this in women suggests that when women direct their aggression towards others their victims are generally those within their domestic sphere of control – a partner, a family member, a child, a friend, a work colleague. This may involve the manipulation of or damage to peer relationships. Thus they use aggressive competitiveness, the withdrawal of friendship, ostracism, overt bullying, and lie about their victims to promote their rejection by others and exclusion from the social group. Conversely, when men direct their aggression towards others its function is to damage their victims' sense of control or dominance over the perpetrator. Male aggression is more visible than female aggression and more likely to result in arrest and punishment. Sociopathy in particular and antisocial behaviour in general in women has been subject to little systematic investigation. Furthermore the harmful potential of some sociopathic women can be overlooked, as in this case in the workplace but especially towards partners and children.

The sociopath's standard mode of operation in relationships

In relationships sociopaths often employ additional tactics. There are thought to be three different stages that the abuser leads the relationship through: idealization; devaluation; discarding.

Idealization

During this early stage sociopaths show themselves in the best possible light. In the context of a new romantic relationship the targeted person may feel intense love for the sociopath. Caught up in the euphoria, the target becomes hooked. In the context of friendship, targets can have feelings of having found someone with whom they have more in common than with anyone they have ever met. In the workplace they have finally found a boss who sees their true potential. The target does everything possible to gain special approval.

Devaluation

Once the sociopath has assessed the target's strengths and weaknesses, it is time for the devaluation stage to begin. From here on the sociopath is cold and unfeeling. At some point the partner or friend or family member will feel unable to do anything right. They feel devalued at every turn. Totally confused, the sociopath's target becomes increasingly stressed, unhappy, low in mood or depressed. The gaslighting effect – see overleaf – is underway. Confused, the targeted person tries harder to please the sociopathic abuser in order to get the relationship back on track. Targets get caught up in spiralling sociopathic abuse where unpredictability and uncertainty become routine, until finally they become shadows of their former selves. Devaluation can be delivered through many different forms and levels of attack.

Discarding

In this phase the game comes to its close. By this time the sociopath has lost ardour for the game, viewing it as an already won contest. The targeted person is reduced to an object, a 'something' to which the sociopath is totally indifferent. The target is left confused and raw with emotion while the sociopath resists all attempts to re-establish any connection, using bullying tactics such as silence or coldness in retaliation, and is likely to be making moves to secure his or her next target.

Sociopaths and other antisocialites use manipulation as a means to control or as a way to abuse other people. One tried and tested tactic they frequently use is **gaslighting**. This is the systematic attempt by one person to erode another's reality, and the term gets its name from the 1938 stage play *Gas Light*. The 1944 film adaptation features a murderer who attempts to make his wife doubt her sanity so that she won't be believed when she reports strange things that are actually occurring. One of the tricks he uses to make her feel she is going crazy is to dim the normally unused gas lamps in the attic (where he conducts clandestine activities), yet convinces her no one is up there. The term has since found its way into clinical and research literature.

The effects of gaslighting can be profound. Dr Robin Stern, a psychologist, describes three stages the targeted person goes through: disbelief; defence; depression. At first all that targets know is that something terribly distressing seems to be happening, but they can't work out what it is. Their confidence is so eroded that they can't trust their own view of themselves or the events going on around them. Becoming bewildered and unable to trust their own instincts or indeed their own recollection of events, they tend to isolate themselves owing to the shame they feel. Eventually they succumb to the gaslighting effect. They feel that they can't do anything right any more, don't feel they can trust their own mind or the opinion of others and withdraw into a distorted reality of what is really taking place.

Can sociopaths change their behaviour?

Sociopaths and those others with zero or extremely limited empathy probably have the most fixed natures of everyone on the empathy spectrum. Certainly they seem remarkably resistant to changing their ways. They are good at faking transformation but unlikely to undergo any genuine or long-lasting change. As we said previously, it is probably best, at least while there are no effective means of treatment, to view the sociopath with dispassion and instead use your time and energies to step away from the person with whom you have a traumatic relationship to avoid ending up an object of abuse. Of paramount importance is being aware of the sociopath's more unscrupulous personality traits. After that it is a matter of learning how best to take care of yourself so as to avoid abuse. In

Chapter 4 we look at what it takes to deal with sociopaths in the family and how to instigate boundaries when communicating and interacting with them. We also address the issue of severing all ties if they pose a serious risk to your lasting well-being.

Borderline personality traits

The term 'borderline personality' was proposed by Adolph Stern in the USA in 1938. Stern introduced the term to describe what he observed, which is that the condition 'bordered' on other conditions. People with a borderline personality disorder (BPD) have a serious problem that affects their intimate, personal and family relationships. In Chapter 2 we presented Megan (see p. 14), who has BPD, except that in her situation, and as is often the case, the disorder goes undiagnosed. This is the usual state of affairs and one that often leaves people with BPD traits and their families without the know-how or support to deal with the problems that manifest.

Borderline personality disorder is thought to affect less than 1 per cent of the population. It is a condition that is usually diagnosed only in adults and it is estimated that three-quarters of those given the diagnosis are women. As a result of its position on the 'border' of other conditions, BPD is often diagnosed alongside depression and anxiety, eating disorders such as bulimia, post-traumatic stress disorder (PTSD), substance-use disorders and bipolar disorder, a condition characterized by severe swings in mood with which BPD is sometimes clinically confused.

The causes of BPD are unclear. Most researchers think that it develops through a combination of factors, including temperament and childhood and adolescent experiences. Difficult life events such as the early loss of a parent, childhood neglect and sexual or physical abuse are common in people diagnosed with BPD, though this is not always the case. Stressful experiences, such as the break-up of a relationship or the loss of a job, can lead to already present symptoms of BPD getting worse.

BPD can cause a wide range of symptoms, which can be broadly divided into four main areas: emotional instability; disturbed patterns of thinking or perception; impulsive behaviour; intense but unstable relationships.

Emotional instability

According to NHS Choices, the UK's biggest health website (see the Useful addresses section), if you have BPD you may experience a range of often intense negative emotions, such as rage, shame, panic and terror. Individuals with BPD may also experience long-term feelings of emptiness and loneliness. They may also have severe mood swings over a short space of time. It is common for people with BPD to feel suicidal with despair and then fairly positive a few hours later. The pattern varies, but the key sign is that moods swing in unpredictable ways.

Disturbed patterns of thinking or perception

People with BPD can have upsetting thoughts, such as thinking they are terrible people or wishing they didn't exist. They may seek reassurance from others that these thoughts are not true. They may also have brief episodes of abnormal experiences, such as hearing voices that may instruct them to harm themselves or others (they may or may not know whether these are real). Furthermore they may have prolonged episodes of unusual experiences, such as hallucinations (voices outside their heads talking to them) and distressing beliefs (believing, for example, that their family are secretly trying to kill them). These beliefs may be delusions and a sign that they are becoming more unwell. It is important to encourage people struggling with delusions to get professional medical help because of the overlap with psychotic disorders – severe mental disorders that cause abnormal thinking and perceptions. The overlap between BPD and the more severe mental disorders like schizophrenia can be considerable. Schizophrenia is an example of a psychotic disorder. These disorders involve distorted awareness and thinking. Two of the most common symptoms are hallucinations – the experience of images or sounds that are not real, such as hearing voices – and delusions, which are false beliefs that the ill person accepts as true despite evidence to the contrary. The difference between schizophrenia and BPD in our context is that in BPD the delusions are usually brief and linked to times of extreme emotional instability. The brevity distinguishes the symptoms from those of schizophrenia and related psychotic disorders.

Impulsive behaviour

There are two main types of impulses that individuals may find extremely difficult to control. The first is an impulse to self-harm, such as cutting their arms with razors or burning their skin with cigarettes. In severe cases, especially if they feel so intensely sad and depressed, this impulse can lead to feeling suicidal or attempting suicide. The second impulse is a strong urge to engage in reckless activities, such as binge drinking, drug abuse, going on an excessive spending spree or having unprotected sex with strangers. Impulsive behaviours are especially dangerous when people are in brief deluded states because they are much more likely to act impulsively if their judgement is impaired.

Intense but unstable relationships

People with BPD also tend to have unstable relationships. They may feel that other people abandon them when they most need them, or conversely find their friendships smothering. Mostly they swing between these positions. The fear of abandonment can lead to feelings of intense anxiety and anger and result in frantic efforts, including constant texting or phoning, in a bid to prevent being left alone. They may suddenly call a friend or family member in the middle of the night or cling to that person and refuse to let go, or they may make threats that they will harm or kill themselves if that person ever leaves them.

Fear of being smothered or controlled provokes intense fear and anger. People with BPD may respond by acting in ways to make others go away, such as emotionally withdrawing from, rejecting or verbally abusing them. Not surprisingly these two patterns often result in unstable relations with others. Like the sociopath, the person with BPD is often drawn to empathic and caring individuals because of their understanding and perceptive nature, yet the very rigid black–white view of relationships of the person with BPD often results in swings from viewing the empath as wonderful one minute and viewing him or her as interfering and disagreeable the next. Thus for many individuals with diagnosed or undiagnosed BPD, relationships with other people are confusing and often a source of stress for them and their friends and partners. Sadly this often leads to relationship and friendship break-ups.

Being a relative of someone with BPD can be fraught with emotional difficulty. In the end individuals can become so caught up in the chaos of the person with BPD that they may lose touch with their individuality and their own separate thoughts, feelings, beliefs, opinions and so on. According to Paul Mason and Randi Kreger, the authors of *Stop Walking on Eggshells*, becoming enmeshed in this way is very common in high-conflict relationships, where individuals exhibit behaviour that increases conflict rather than reduces or resolves it. And it's not limited to partners – whole families can become enmeshed.

In contrast, peaceable and empathic personalities may be attracted to putting another's needs before their own, and more willing than most to do so, and so may find themselves caught up in the emotional chaos of the individual with BPD. Regularly exposed to angry outbursts, they may not fare well since empaths tend to feel extremely uncomfortable with conflict. Nevertheless empaths' caring traits make them more prone to take on the mantel of the emotional caretaker in the family, which makes them vulnerable to abuse. Margalis Fjelstad's book *Stop Caretaking the Borderline or Narcissist* deals with this in detail (see Further reading).

Narcissistic personality traits

Narcissistic personality disorder (NPD) is a condition characterized by an inflated sense of self-importance, a need for admiration, extreme self-preoccupation and a lack of empathy for others. Individuals with this disorder are usually arrogantly self-assured and confident. They expect to be treated as superior. Many highly successful individuals might be considered narcissistic. However, the disorder is only diagnosed when these behaviours become persistent, very disabling or distressing. Usually NPD begins to show in early adulthood. Our case example, Bob, is a classic narcissist (see pp. 15–16). He's already destroyed his first marriage with his destructive and self-absorbed characteristics and is well on the way to ruining yet another relationship, the one with his daughter. Bob's neediness and manipulative nature may sometimes get him what he wants but they also put his relationships at risk because his selfishness proves overwhelming. He is what we might call 'interpersonally exploitative', meaning that he uses others to achieve his own ends. He is unable or unwilling to identify with, acknowledge or accept the feelings, needs and choices of others. The case study demonstrates just how little he can comprehend the preferences and feelings of another, in this instance his own daughter. Parental love sets the basis for how you will deal with the world and yourself throughout life, which leaves the child of a narcissist at a disadvantage because narcissistic parents cannot feel love and may dislike affection and intimacy. However, they often draw people in and need people around them and have very specific reasons for being in relationships and having friendships – they are to ensure their needs are met. Narcissists feed off the attention they get from others. They have a need to feel special, to be worshipped and adored, and that is often what fuels and sustains them. Narcissistic tendencies sometimes can be seen in grandparents who are probably merely continuing lifelong patterns and are so intent on living their own lives – second or third marriages, hobbies, cruises – that they are simply not available to the younger generation.

The prevalence of NPD is less than 1 per cent of the UK population. It is seen in 2–16 per cent of psychiatric outpatients and is more frequent in males (50–75 per cent) than females. The range in estimates is large because many people with NPD are misdiagnosed with something else (this is not surprising, given that distinctions between the disorders are blurred and confusing). Furthermore narcissistic traits are very common in adolescents, but most adolescents grow out of this. Narcissistic traits are to some extent limited by our culture, or the reverse can be true and narcissism can be validated by it.

A propensity to low self-esteem makes individuals with NPD very sensitive to criticism or defeat. Although they may not outwardly show it, criticism may leave them feeling humiliated, degraded, hollow and empty. They may react with disdain, rage or defiantly start an offensive. They are frequently envious of others and may even seek to hurt the objects of their frustration. This can lead to danger for partners and children of narcissists, particularly if in extreme and rare circumstances the person with NPD suffers from persecutory (paranoid) delusions.

People like Bob with NPD often find their social life impaired owing to their own conduct. Problems often arise from their sense of entitlement, need for admiration and their relative disregard for the sensitivities of others. Though their excessive ambition and inflated sense of confidence may lead to high achievement, performance may be affected by intolerance of criticism or fear of being defeated or losing out in some way. Sometimes this can lead to an unwillingness to compete or risk other situations where defeat is possible. Individuals with narcissistic traits have special difficulties adjusting to growing old, especially if this is accompanied by a loss of status.

With narcissism, sustained feelings of shame or humiliation can lead to social withdrawal and depressed mood. Surprisingly, sustained periods of grandiosity also may be associated with a low mood. Eating disorders, substance-use disorders (especially stimulants like cocaine) and other personality disorders (especially borderline and antisocial) frequently accompany this disorder and are discussed briefly in Chapters 5 and 6, alongside other behaviours linked to low empathy.

Other antisocialite traits

To complete our review of the antisocialites (we admit this is not an exhaustive account), we pay attention to a final 'group': those who behave in ways similar to sociopaths, narcissists and borderline personalities but whose exact cluster of behaviours do not properly match so cannot be defined, at least in medical terms, as personality disordered. In this group we put passive aggressives and other non-diagnosable personality traits. People in this category may have other accompanying antisocial behaviours – eating and substance-use disorders are quite common. These problems aren't themselves signs of zero or very limited empathy but often accentuate the individual's antisocial traits.

Among antisocialites of all kinds a parasitic nature is commonly observed. People living with a person with strong parasitic tendencies can feel quite literally as though life is being sucked out of them. Passive aggression is one such example. It is a particularly pernicious form of manipulative behaviour. Passive aggressives don't deal with things directly. They talk behind your back and put others in the position of telling you what they won't say themselves; find subtle ways of letting you know they are not happy; are unlikely to show their angry or resentful natures; conceal it behind a façade of affability and politeness and a show of well-meaning. However, underneath manipulation is going on. Types of passive aggression include:

Victimization – a situation where passive aggressives are unable to look at their own part in a situation and turn the tables to become victims, or at least behave like victims.

Self-pity – the 'poor me' kind of scenario, where passive aggressives blame others for situations rather than take responsibility for their own actions; withhold usual behaviours or roles such as sex; sabotage social arrangements to reinforce to other parties that they are angry.

Learned helplessness – where someone has learned to behave helplessly, failing to respond even though there are opportunities to help herself or himself by avoiding unpleasant circumstances.

The important thing to establish is that passive aggression is a destructive pattern of behaviour that can lead to emotional abuse. Such behaviours cause great distress to someone on the receiving end, who may feel overburdened with guilt and responsibility for the passive aggressive person.

In the next chapter we look at these issues from the point of view of those affected by the behaviours of individuals in the family with zero or very low empathy. We consider the importance of instigating boundaries in communication and discuss how to get some sense of personal control back when relations have deteriorated and things look set for disaster.

4

Strategies for coping with antisocialites in the family

In this chapter we explore ways to avoid becoming overwhelmed by the behaviour and actions of antisocialites like George, Laura's mother and Bob. We consider the importance of instigating boundaries in communication and discuss how to get some sense of personal control back when relations have deteriorated and things look set for disaster. Having someone in the family who instigates drama and chaos all the time usually means endless problems and worry for everyone else. Many people in chaotic relationships only realize the relationship is destructive when the dramatic tension hits its height – perhaps they walk out, or you can't take any more of their drama and challenge them in a serious way. As we mentioned in earlier chapters, the most extreme antisocialites like sociopaths, though often quite charming when they want something from you, typically behave badly and most aggressively when you challenge them. It is at the point of challenge or confrontation that antisocialites become their most aggressive and dangerous and can leave you severely traumatized, as discussed in Chapter 3 (the gaslighting process – see p. 34). Here we talk you through strategies for dealing with such situations.

Recovering from the gaslighting process

During the process of gaslighting, the targeted person usually goes through some recognizable emotional and psychological states of mind. Dr Robin Stern, a psychologist, describes three stages: disbelief; defence; depression.

Disbelief

Targeted people's initial reaction to gaslighting behaviour is one of complete disbelief – they cannot believe the sudden change towards them. All they know is that something terribly distressing seems to be happening. Blinded by the promises or affections of the sociopath, targeted people naturally trust that their friendship or love is returned, but of course this belief is based on falsehood. Gaslighting does not need to be severe in order to have stark effects on the gaslighted person. It can be as subtle as being told 'You are so sensitive'. Even though gaslighted people know on a rational level that these statements are untrue, their confidence is so eroded that they can't trust their own judgement. In extreme cases, those desperate for reassurance that they're not going mad become very dependent on their abuser for a sense of reality.

Defence

At some point people on the receiving end of abuse are thrown off balance by creeping self-doubt, anxiety and guilt. Becoming bewildered and unable to trust their own instincts or recollection of events, they tend to isolate themselves because of the shame they feel. One psychological condition that can result is called Stockholm syndrome, where targeted people may bond with their abuser as a defence mechanism. They may rationalize and excuse the sociopath's behaviour in order to reduce the conflict they are experiencing.

Depression

When people have been systematically gaslit, they reach a point where they feel disorientated and hold a distorted view of what is taking place. Most people in this situation experience an array of responses: shock, disbelief, deep sadness, guilt, shame, anger. And many also express relief at finally knowing what has been going on. Shame and blame are the hallmarks of gaslighting.

The good thing to come from this phase in the gaslighting process is that most sociopaths give up manipulating their target at this point – usually because they've already set their sights on a new one!

The importance of taking control of the situation

You need to be firm in your dealings with sociopaths and learn to instigate boundaries to block the worst effects of their persistent games. If you think the antisocial person in your life is potentially dangerous, and you perceive that you, some other adult or children are at risk, you should seek help from the authorities – the police, social services – and take legal advice.

The important thing if you have been gaslit is to recognize that it has happened. Talk to friends, read books, look online, or in an even more severe situation, attend counselling or therapy.

Setting boundaries

Limiting contact is one step you can take to protect you and your loved ones, and in many circumstances it is probably best to have no contact at all. This is a challenge when you are dealing with someone who has no regard for your personal safety or welfare. It becomes even more of a challenge when children are involved.

When children are involved

Those who have children with an antisocialite will have to spell out the boundaries to avoid further conflict. It is hard to accept the uncomfortable truth that sociopaths and narcissistic types and others with hardly any empathy don't love their children for themselves but as objects to manipulate.

Sociopaths and narcissistic types are often indifferent to the welfare of children. This indifference may take many forms. They may leave young children alone or in the care of unreliable babysitters or neglect them, for instance by failing to provide proper food and clothing. They may demand certain behaviour or accomplishments for their own benefit or that they can revel in. They may inflict physical and emotional abuse, or expose a child to inappropriate or dangerous activities. So when sociopaths are involved with children, always be on guard.

A non-sociopathic parent can thus be dealt a double blow at the hands of a former partner, experiencing secondary trauma whenever children or other loved ones are involved, so look for the patterns of behaviour. Don't behave apathetically – open your eyes! If you witness abuse, do something about it, and if you have been abused yourself and you can see this now, have some self-compassion and do what you need to do to protect yourself. Our earlier book, *The Empathy Trap*, focuses in particular on the complexities of sociopaths and sociopathy in families, but we also provide information about support available in difficult situations in the Useful addresses at the end of this book.

Different countries have different laws governing the protection and safeguarding of children, but in the UK there is a comprehensive child welfare system under which local authorities have duties towards children in need in their area. Risk of 'significant harm' to children covers physical, sexual and emotional abuse and neglect. The basic legal principle in the UK, under the Children Act of 1989, is that the welfare of the child is paramount.

For those who have no option but to remain in contact with an extreme antisocial person, boundaries are of the utmost importance. Metaphorically speaking it is best not to erect a high brick wall behind which to barricade yourself. The better option is to imagine the boundary as a low and sturdy fence, something you can still communicate over. Boundaries in your communications and interactions should stop the other person invading your personal space. It's all about learning to have relationships on your terms, and developing more self-compassion – the ability to stand back from and understand your own thoughts and feelings.

Severing ties completely

While it can be relatively straightforward to cut ties with a person who is fairly new in your life or just a familiar face in your social group, a relationship that has been intimate and long-standing is often more complicated. A mother may feel unnatural severing ties with her child, even if that child is a full-grown adult with antisocial tendencies! Likewise an adult child may feel a sense of abandonment or that he or she will be perceived as unnatural or ungrateful for turning away from a narcissistic parent or sibling. It can take years to work towards separation because intense emotions can so readily upend the decision-making process. The important message to take on board is that you are not responsible for the other person's behaviour, but you are bound to act morally in ways that safeguard your own welfare and that of any children.

If you do cut ties there are issues to consider, such as ensuring other friends and acquaintances do not play 'go between'. You will need to make it clear that you do not want to discuss anything about the person or people with whom you have permanently ceased contact. If the third party refuses to respect your wishes you should consider limiting contact with them as well.

Cutting ties with an antisocialite who is abusive and dangerous is a painful and terminal step, but it is often necessary because a lot of the personality types we are talking about here have conditions that are both treatment and punishment insensitive, which means nothing can be done to make them reform their ways (at least this is the situation we face at present). It takes time to absorb the fact that there is nothing that can be done to make them see things your way or care about how their actions are viewed from your perspective, and that guilt-tripping them is entirely counterproductive as they've no conscience to work on and get through to. At some point you will realize that the only worthwhile thing to do is leave them to their unending games and take steps to liberate yourself from the whole sorry situation.

Making a clean break from a destructive relationship or friendship involves permanently cutting ties. You will need to block the person from contacting you, whether by telephone or social media. Don't accept gifts – they are likely to be an attempt to manipulate you. Likewise don't respond to letters or emails but do keep their communiqués in case you need them as legal evidence. Do not enter into dialogue as it is best to give no energy or stimulus at all. With luck the person will soon tire of attempts to woo you back and move on to someone else.

Overcoming emotional trauma

Shame and guilt after a trauma or abuse often persist. Paul Gilbert, the originator of compassion focused therapy, suggests that we have at least three types of emotion-regulation systems: threat detection and protection; drive and excitement; contentment and soothing – the latter making us want to go to our nearest and dearest when under threat because we have an intuitive wisdom that the kindness of others is what helps and what soothes us and restores a sense of safety. Hence in trying to help yourself or someone else get over the trauma of sociopathic abuse it is important to have your fears and painful experiences validated by someone else. Who hears you out is for you to decide, but we call this person an 'enlightened witness', a term coined by the author and child-abuse expert Alice

Miller to describe people willing to support harmed individuals and help them gain understanding of their past and recent experiences. An enlightened person could be someone, such as a relative or friend, who already knows you and will understand your situation, or a trained therapist.

Your early life experiences, such as being bullied, particularly if you are the adult child of an antisocial parent, may have sensitized your threat system, and emotional memories can lead to 'safety strategies' – such as avoiding confrontation with others or engaging in people-pleasing behaviour – that can end up lowering your self-esteem and increasing your vulnerability to anxiety and depression. Normal defensive emotions may also be feared, such as expressing anger, so fear of emotion is important to explore and may require you to consider undergoing trauma therapy.

Once you've found some source of comfort and put some initial boundaries in place, you will also need to be consistent in your new approach to the other person. And that means becoming trigger savvy! A trigger is something you associate with something or someone else that you are inclined to respond to. Years of conditioning mean that a particular trigger will set off a reaction in you by a process of association, much in the way a ringing bell will trigger in a dog the same response as food. Triggers can be either 'hot' or 'cold'. A **hot trigger** is something that affects you immediately – someone yelling at you, demanding something of you, or being stuck in a traffic jam. A **cold trigger** is something that affects you indirectly – watching something on television that reminds you of a situation you've been in with the antisocialite, or listening to some music that reminds you of better times with your difficult partner. A hot trigger forces an immediate response while a cold trigger builds up over time. Triggers work as a call to action and can cause us to act on impulse. To avoid lapsing back to previous behaviour it helps to find a way to disconnect our feelings from the object of association.

The steps to breaking the connections involve looking for patterns. First we need to see clearly the things that make us think about the person we have removed from our lives. Once we recognize the kind of thing that brings them to mind and discover what things act as hot or cold triggers, it is useful to a make a mental or even written note of them.

You will need to analyse your own scenarios/triggers and devise ways to break the associations. Maybe just being aware that a trigger can arouse unwanted feelings and memories is enough. Perhaps you need to talk yourself out of reacting whenever a trigger arrives uninvited. Understanding how best to dampen the effects of emerging triggers is important in behaviour change.

> Ben had not been in contact with his sociopathic brother for six months when a text arrived. He recognized this as a hot trigger, and knew that if he opened the text he would be in a high risk situation, that is, in danger of contacting him back. This was a risky position for Ben because his brother was very manipulative and the situation could put him at risk of lapsing into regular contact, an injurious situation for him. Because he recognized the position he was in and had thought what would be his response if this happened, he was able calmly to delete the message and get back on with his day, as opposed to getting more agitated. Being trigger savvy led to a high risk situation being avoided.

Advice about dealing with individuals with borderline personalities

In her book *Stop Caretaking the Borderline or Narcissist*, Margalis Fjelstad describes how people get into a caretaker role with someone with borderline or narcissistic personality disorder. According to Fjelstad, caretakers give up their sense of self to become who and what the person with BPD or NPD needs them to be. This affects caretakers' self-esteem and distorts their thinking. At worst it locks them into a victim–persecutor–rescuer pattern of behaviour. Caretakers need to move themselves out of these rigid interactions and into a healthier and more positive way of being and interacting. That new way of being can be with or without the BPD or NPD partner or family member. Being more self-focused on their own wants, needs and life goals permits people with BPD or NPD to take care of themselves. This is the best and most compassionate attitude and response to have towards these sorts of relationships.

In another book about borderline personalities, *Stop Walking on Eggshells*, Paul Mason and Randi Kreger suggest that the trouble for those taking care of individuals with BPD occurs when time passes and caretakers stop taking care of their own needs. Their own thoughts, feelings, beliefs, opinions, hobbies and life become enmeshed with the other person's. It's not limited to parents or partners – whole families can be enmeshed. Like so many things, enmeshment is something that exists in the mind. Your attitudes and beliefs will determine whether you are willing to continue to permit enmeshment in your relationship or not. If you continue to think that enmeshment is normal and is the usual way to show or prove your love, you will continue to be in enmeshed relationships. Once you have become aware of your attitude and beliefs in this area and the stranglehold enmeshment has on you, you'll be in a better position to change it.

If the person you are concerned about sometimes or frequently self-harms, it is important for him or her to understand that this behaviour has consequences. Here are some things that are worth doing if the person with BPD threatens or actually commits self-harm.

- If the person harms themselves (or others), notify the person's GP or the out-of-hours service. In emergencies dial 999. If you live outside of the UK, contact your emergency medical services.
- Since self-harm usually occurs when the individual with BPD feels out of control, don't add to that person's turmoil by being in a panic yourself.
- Help the person with BPD organize a care team, and ask him or her to keep its contact details to hand and to get in touch at the least concern about his or her behaviour.
- Emphasize that you care about the person but wish she or he would find another way of dealing with her or his problems.
- Try and stress the improvements, even little steps forward, such as not self-harming for a longer period than usual.
- Suggest alternative, less harmful alternative actions – see if the person can identify other activities that produce a strong sensation that is not harmful (strenuous exercise, for example). But do let the person identify the alternative as you can't force people to adopt new strategies for coping.
- Refuse to be put in a compromised situation, such as promising not to seek help because the person is embarrassed or ashamed. Don't agree to keep the self-harming a secret between you. Tell the person you are not qualified to handle the situation on your own, and it is unreasonable to be asked to keep this to yourself.

- Most importantly, if you start to feel overwhelmed by the person's behaviour and self-harming, step back. You may have overestimated his or her reliance on you, and at any rate, it is unhealthy to think that you are the person to bring about a fix. That ultimately rests with the person.

General advice for dealing with antisocialites

The best defence against antisocial behaviour is to increase your perspective-taking abilities. It's no use to anyone if you turn a blind eye to potential or actual abusive situations and offer no assistance to anyone, including yourself, or if you are apathetic and sit on the fence.

- Prevent antisocial types getting the upper hand by confronting not only your own apathy but that of those around you. Tell partners, or whatever family members are self-harming, about the strengths you witness in them, the moments when you have worried that they weren't being true to themselves and the challenges you think they need to overcome.
- State your opinions and learn to take sides. Don't go along to get along. Genuine beliefs, duly considered and powerfully presented, are insulation against apathy. Empathy is not for the faint hearted – expressing views about the world and showing compassion for the people in it takes courage.
- Encourage others to say what they think and believe too. Listen attentively to their answers, then ask a few questions designed to help them to dig deeper into their thoughts and feelings.
- Learn anger control – people who exhibit aggressive behaviour at home need to learn anger control. There are a number of cognitive and behavioural techniques that trained counsellors and therapists can teach individuals with conditions like BPD. One such is **brief strategic family therapy**, the main elements of which include engaging and supporting the family, identifying maladaptive family interactions and seeking to promote new and more adaptive family interactions. You can find out more about the therapy options available from your doctor.
- In relation to people with BPD and those who exhibit similar or less disturbing behaviours, other skills such as relaxation and

social skills may also be taught if the person is referred to a qualified and experienced therapist.

- Unfortunately sociopaths and psychopaths and others with extreme antisocial tendencies are most often unresponsive to both therapeutic treatment and punishment. In situations such as these, therefore, the best approach is *not* to approach but to instigate boundaries in relation to communications and interaction or limit or cease contact.

- Practise more self-love! Loving yourself means valuing yourself. Practising aloneness can prove a self-valuing activity, so respect each other's need for solitude. This applies to all manner of relationships – learning to be comfortable when alone helps us let go of unhealthy enmeshments and attachments.

In the next chapter we turn our attentions to those in the family who may not be aware of it – even if you are! – but who have problems related to low empathy.

5

Personalities of low empathy

Do you have a sibling like Michaela, whom we met in Chapter 1, someone who is moody, blames others and is rather dispirited about life? Do you have a family member who seems aloof or rather detached? Is that person unsociable and/or uncommunicative? Have you noticed tendencies like John's, from our case study of undiagnosed Asperger syndrome (AS) in Chapter 2 (see p. 19)? Does he or she seem extremely preoccupied with things, have obsessive habits or engage in activities that require spending inordinate amounts of time away from you and the family (at a pub, betting shop or on the internet)? One of the underlying issues here could be low empathy.

In this chapter we introduce people with low empathy and invite you to utilize your powers of empathy to make sense of the world of social interaction as it's experienced by them. Because their chances of moving along the empathy spectrum are less restricted than the antisocialite group, we focus on the small changes – the bit-by-bit changes – that can help improve family interrelations. We include in this category personalities on the autistic spectrum specifically, AS, and those with obsessive traits, for instance obsessive–compulsive disorders, addiction problems and other entrenched behaviours.

Autistic spectrum disorders

Autism and related conditions involve impaired cognitive empathy (being able to read what other people are thinking) and emotional empathy (responding with an appropriate emotion to another's mental state). The exact causes of autism are unknown. The National Autistic Society says there are over half a million people in the UK with autism – that is around 1 in 100. Because there is a wide range of severity and symptoms, the conditions are collectively known as **autistic spectrum disorders** (ASDs). Due to the fluctuating and imprecise criteria for the diagnosis of ASDs, even a formal diagnosis cannot be taken as certain proof that a given person is on the spectrum, and self-diagnosis of AS is common.

Autism is considered to be a neurological disorder. The National Autistic Society states that there is evidence to suggest that genetic factors are responsible for some forms of autism. However, as in the case of sociopathy and its variants, the difficulty of establishing gene involvement is compounded by the interaction of genes and the way they combine with environmental factors. Various studies over the years have sought to identify potential genes, so far inconclusively. Nevertheless a new study by Jordan Smoller and colleagues, published in 2013 in the medical journal *The Lancet*, suggests that five distinct psychiatric disorders – autism, attention-deficit/hyperactivity disorder (ADHD), bipolar disorder, major depressive disorder and schizophrenia – may share some genetic risk factors (Smoller et al. 2013). These findings confirm what many researchers already thought – that genetic risk factors aren't necessarily specific to one disease.

People with ASDs don't always show the appropriate emotions in response to other people's feelings. And other people often don't realize that autistic people don't display empathy in the usual way – instead they assume they are being rude! However, people with ASDs are often more affected by the situation than they appear to be – they just don't know how to express interest or concern appropriately. Because of their apparent rudeness or aloofness, people with ASDs are often confused with those with conditions like sociopathy. However, the social problems of people on the autistic spectrum and those of antisocialites are not just different, they are almost opposite. For where the sociopath often understands what others are thinking but doesn't feel for them, people with ASDs often have a keen sense of morality and care deeply for others, though they do not always demonstrate empathy in the ways society expects.

Autism and related conditions affect how people communicate with and relate to other people. They also affect how they make sense of the world around them. People on the autistic spectrum may find it difficult to tell others what they need and how they feel; may not speak, and use things like pictures or sign language to communicate; may not understand – or may copy – what other people say or do; may only talk about their favourite subject and do the same activity every day; may be very interested in one thing and know a lot about it; may also be good at remembering information.

While all people with autistic traits share certain difficulties, their conditions will affect them in different ways. Some are able to live relatively independent lives but others may have accompanying learning disabilities and need a lifetime of specialist support. Some may also experience over- or undersensitivity to sounds, touch, tastes, smells, light or colours. And probably the hardest thing to deal with is that their particular difficulties are often poorly understood by other people.

The problem for people with ASDs, diagnosed or not, is that their behaviour and ways of being are often perplexing to everyone else. Those who don't share the same view of the world can find their behaviour deeply vexing. But the reality is that people with ASDs can, and often do, behave and operate in ways that benefit others. In other words they can be as prosocial – cooperative and considerate of others – as people higher up the empathy spectrum. Nowadays we tend not to talk of seeking a 'cure' for ASDs. It is important to celebrate the difference and look to the considerable benefits people with ASDs can bring to society. For example, they can be immensely focused in their work and other endeavours, including working on ideas and resources that contribute to the public good. It is thought that Albert Einstein would have fitted the criteria for AS had he been born at a time when it was a recognized and diagnosable condition.

The autism expert Simon Baron-Cohen suggests that the trait that marks people with Asperger out is their particular cognitive style – being attentive to details and patterns or rules. He calls this 'systemizing', as mentioned in Chapter 2. Systemizing can have very positive consequences for the individual and for society, though there is of course a downside – some areas of life are resistant to systemizing efforts, for example other people and their emotions!

Asperger syndrome

We single out AS, sometimes called high-functioning autism, from the group of conditions on the autistic spectrum because it is the most common of the disorders and yet underdiagnosed. There is no register of people with autism or AS in the UK, so it is hard to know the actual prevalence of the condition. However, estimates suggest 1 per 1,000 adults has AS, and some experts argue that it could be as high as 1 in 300. It is thought to be at least ten times more common in men than women. Symptoms vary from so mild that the person can function as well as anyone else, to so severe that he or she is completely unable to take part in normal society.

In brief, AS in adults is characterized by problems of social interaction and communication. Individuals often exhibit distinct patterns of behaviour and may have a narrow repertoire of interests upon which they very keenly and intensely focus. It is a condition that emerges in childhood and remains present throughout life to varying degrees. Some people may have AS traits but not be diagnosed with AS.

Asperger syndrome was defined in 1944 by Hans Asperger but only included in the WHO's International Classification of Diseases (ICD) in 1992, and in the American Psychiatric Association's manual of mental disorders in 1994. In May 2013 the latest version of the Diagnostic and Statistical Manual of Mental Disorders (DSM-V), which we have encountered more than once, discarded the label Asperger: as we noted in Chapter 2, the single diagnostic label of autistic spectrum disorder now serves for all. The DSM is very influential, although the main set of criteria used in the UK is the ICD. The next version, ICD-11, is due to be published in 2015, and though it could also drop the diagnosis label Asperger, the descriptions in ICD are slightly different from the American Psychiatric Association's and are likely to remain so. Those currently diagnosed with AS should expect to remain diagnosed whether it is decided to continue to use the term AS or ASD. In truth, many doctors are likely to continue to use the term for some years to come and those currently holding an AS diagnosis condition will continue to be recognized.

Twenty years ago there was little public awareness of AS, yet as awareness has increased, people with these traits are becoming increasingly visible in the mainstream, including television and other media. Sheldon Cooper, a character in the US television comedy series *The Big Bang Theory*, exemplifies this changed situation. That said, the AS character has been known for centuries in all but name, as is evident in literature. Characterization in literature – the art of enlarging the psychological makeup of characters so that they become recognizable personalities – alerts us to the fact that the autistic character was known about in times past. For example, Sir Arthur Conan Doyle's character Sherlock Holmes apparently had at least two character traits that typify AS: his keen power of analysis and deduction; his indifference to the more emotional aspects of human nature.

Undiagnosed AS in adults

There are an estimated 225,000 adults living with AS in the UK, most of whom don't know they have it because they get by and hold down jobs. In August 2013, in an article in the *Daily Mail* entitled 'Husband a right old grump?', the journalist Anna Magee challenged the newspaper's female readers to consider whether their partner could be one of thousands of men who have AS without realizing it. The article featured a man, not unlike John from our case study in Chapter 2 (see p. 19), who had undiagnosed AS. Like John, the character of the man in the newspaper article loved detail, order and lists. He also had an anger problem, which stemmed from triggers at home and at work activating high levels of stress and anxiety.

In Britain AS was only recognized in 1994. As a result it is likely that the vast majority of undiagnosed adult autism cases are those with AS who grew up before the disorder was identified. On top of that, and according to a recent report by the National Audit Office in which eight out of ten doctors admitted they didn't have enough knowledge or training in autism, adults with AS often slip through the net. Individuals may avoid diagnosis because they don't seek a diagnosis for their character and way of being, or their symptoms are subtle and get missed. In either case it doesn't mean they're not secretly struggling to make sense of their social worlds. People can develop depression and suffer anxiety attacks or find they have used up so much energy trying to act normally that they end up exhausted.

One fairly common problem individuals with AS experience is anger and frustration. Because AS in adults is largely undiagnosed, many people living with someone with the condition may be unaware of it, and suffering rows that could have been avoided in consequence. People with AS often struggle with emotional displays, so their partners frequently interpret their behaviour as uncaring and undemonstrative. They may find it important to stick to their tried and tested plans and routines, and often become upset when others want to do something spontaneous. In our case study we pointed out how John's wife Anne struggled with his rigid and excessively orderly ways. She also found it difficult to cope with his behaviour in social situations, where he often seemed acutely awkward.

Gender differences and AS

The ratio of men to women with AS is not known for certain, and estimates range from 2:1 to 16:1. Because of the gender bias in childhood (the time when AS is most likely to be formally diagnosed), girls are less likely to be diagnosed than boys even when their symptoms are equally severe. According to Tony Attwood, a leading expert in the field of AS, girls are more able to follow social actions by delayed imitation because they observe other children and copy them, perhaps masking the symptoms of AS (Attwood et al. 2006). Nevertheless the National Autistic Society published a paper in 2011 outlining the differences in the way AS manifests in girls and women. Some differences in social interaction are observed in women with AS. In general women are often more aware of, and feel, a need to interact socially, and are expected to be social in their communication. Girls and women on the autistic spectrum do not do social 'chit chat' in order to facilitate social communication in the same way as other women. In addition, how one communicates with people of different status can be problematic and can get girls with AS into trouble with teachers and women into trouble with employers. However, the interests of girls and women in the spectrum are very often similar to other girls and women. It is not the special interests that differentiate them from their peers but the quality and intensity of these interests. In women AS also commonly manifests as passive or anxious behaviour; thus it is sometimes confused with conditions like obsessive–compulsive disorder or other entrenched behaviour problems such as eating disorders.

Being a partner or spouse of someone with AS

Being the partner or spouse can be very difficult for the person with AS and vice versa, especially if the disorder goes unrecognized. Although people with AS are very capable of being in love and intimately sharing their lives with others, their traits can put them at a disadvantage in relationships. In her book *Asperger Syndrome in Adults*, Dr Ruth Searle suggests that a man with AS is often attracted to his prospective partner largely because she or he finds him attractive or likes him. This is based on the man's need for approval and to be needed, following a lifetime of rejection and disapproval. Whether or not the relationship lasts may depend on how adaptable his partner is, for he is unlikely to find it easy to adapt to the other person's needs and wants. Once in a relationship he is more likely to drop his guard and in doing so, his rigid behaviour and beliefs are likely to be revealed.

Other issues associated with low empathy

Eating disorders

Eating disorders and other obsessive and entrenched behaviours don't just appear out of nowhere. These behaviours are usually a response to deeper emotional pain, depression, anxiety and other interpersonal experiences. Researchers at the Maudsley Hospital in London carried out a study in which autism and anorexia were compared and contrasted (Hambrook et al. 2008). The study found that individuals on the autistic spectrum struggle to connect with people in the outside world whereas anorexics are obsessed with other people's perceptions of them – nevertheless there are still some compelling similarities between the two conditions. Tony Attwood and others writing in this area argue that early ritualistic behaviour around food can be the precursor to having an eating disorder (Attwood et al. 2006). Societal pressure for girls and women to be thin is unhelpful and only adds to the psychological burden. Both men and women with AS tend to be perfectionists, and this perfectionism can apply to the issue of body image. Eating disorders within the autism population can manifest at any time, and it is important to realize that people on the autistic spectrum are not immune to this problematic issue.

Specific personality disorders may put people at higher risk of eating disorders – these include borderline personality disorder, discussed in the previous two chapters, which is associated with self-destructive, impulsive behaviours and narcissistic personalities. Studies have found that people with bulimia or anorexia are often highly narcissistic and self-absorbed. Additionally many people with eating disorders experience depression and anxiety disorders. Depression, anxiety or both are common in families of individuals with eating disorders. It is not clear if emotional disorders, particularly obsessive–compulsive disorder, cause the eating disorders, increase susceptibility to them or share some common biologic and/or environmental cause.

Obsessive–compulsive disorder

Both autism and obsessive–compulsive disorder (OCD) are characterized by obsessions and compulsions. Obsessions are thoughts that on a regular basis plague the individual, while compulsions are behaviours that are repeated over and over again and may be triggered by a certain action or experience. Usually compulsions are automatic and unconscious in people on the autistic spectrum, while OCD compulsions generally are brought on by obsessions. For example, some people with autism might constantly wave their hands about, apparently unaware that they are doing it, while some OCD patients will deliberately wash their hands exactly the same number of times each day.

It is thought that OCD is often a response to life experiences. A trauma in one's life might trigger it as a way to deal with stress and anxiety, which is not the case in autism, which is thought to be present from birth even if symptoms might not become clear for several years. Another difference between people diagnosed with OCD and those known to have an ASD is that people with autism often suffer from **internalized obsessions**, while those with OCD usually suffer from **external obsessions**. For example, some people with AS might be obsessed with washing their hands a specific number of times because they find the repetition somehow reassuring, while some people with OCD might wash obsessively for fear of becoming contaminated with germs.

Sometimes OCD involves the impairment of emotional awareness and perception, which can mean that people with OCD may experience an inability to shift naturally from obsessive thoughts to thoughts about other people in social situations. The social implications of autism and OCD are usually different though. Someone with autism or AS may bond with only a few people over the course of their lives, and sometimes experience rejection from others. People who have OCD, however, may not experience problems making and sustaining relationships, although they may be troubled with paranoia and discomfort if they try to conceal their obsessional behaviour, which in turn can complicate social interaction.

Addiction

Obviously, many people drink alcohol, use drugs, gamble or indulge in other potentially destructive behaviours, but not everyone becomes engrossed in the activity to the point of obsession or addiction. Addiction is often viewed as a problem that takes over all aspects of someone's life – emotionally, behaviourally, socially – and involves an apparent blindness to the harms of the addictive behaviour to oneself and others. Addiction is a complex issue and the causes of it – arguably manifold – remain unresolved.

Some consider that those with addiction problems lack empathy. One of the chief complaints of other family members is that addicted individuals no longer care. They can become completely self-consumed and lose all regard for other people's thoughts and feelings, even those closest to them. People with chronic addiction problems often struggle to identify even their own feelings, let alone the feelings of other people. A psychological syndrome called **alexithymia**, which is the inability to identify and describe one's own feelings, occurs quite commonly in people who chronically use mood-altering substances. Because of this, the development of skills of empathy is often a central theme in the recovery process.

So does addiction or lack of empathy come first? Research rather confusingly points in both directions. There is evidence from studies of children who later developed chronic addiction problems that loss of empathy in many cases preceded their drug use. There's also evidence that this loss of empathy is made worse by becoming heavily reliant upon alcohol and other drugs. Some experts regard the obsessive aspect of addiction as the problem, viewing it as a block on individuals seeing and understanding the emotional needs of others. Dr David Sack, a specialist psychiatrist, calls this 'addiction hijacking empathy' (Sack 2011).

Compounding the issue, addiction is sometimes associated with personality disorders like sociopathy and antisocial personality disorder (AsPD). While most addicts are not sociopaths, many sociopaths do become addicted to activities such as drug-taking or gambling. This is because those with zero empathy and limited emotional repertoire (sociopaths) tend to be drawn towards risky behaviour, which then leads them to activities like criminality and addiction. It can be difficult to get risk-seeking individuals like sociopaths and other antisocialites to seek help for their addiction problems. And even then, once in treatment, though they might break away from addiction, few receive treatment for their AsPD. However, the reverse situation may be true for addicted individuals who don't have an underlying AsPD. In such cases addiction may well be a way of escaping their own remorse or shortcomings or highly empathic natures – problems that sociopaths do not have.

Common psychiatric conditions

Individuals with schizophrenia, bipolar disorder or depression may be less empathic, according to a German study published in the journal *Schizophrenia Research* in late 2012 (Derntl et al. 2012). In the study participants were assessed for responsiveness to various emotion-provoking real-life situations. It suggests that the severity of empathic impairment varies among the different psychiatric conditions. For example, where symptoms of depression dominate, a person tends to obscure the outside world and the people in it. Also people with depression or schizophrenia often describe themselves as feeling emotionally empty (in medical terminology this is sometimes called **anhedonia**, a word derived from Greek meaning 'without pleasure'). Individuals may take the view that others' lives are far happier than their own, and envy them or try to avoid other people; or they may become highly dependent and look to others as caretakers to rescue them.

In bipolar disorder, where states of hopelessness alternate with manic highs, a similar situation is often found, where it can be hard for the individual to empathize deeply with another person's pain. The opposite may be true with anxiety disorders, when an individual's own emotions often feel threatening, and other people's feelings may become overwhelming. Thus people who are extremely anxious are less able or willing to empathize because when they do they can't bear the way they feel inside. This is a problem anxious people share with extreme-end empaths, or super-empaths, who have almost unstoppable powers of empathy and feel too much (see Chapters 10 and 11). In such cases, and as a last resort, people may exit the social realm and become reclusive.

Brain injury

Severe traumatic brain injury (TBI) can leave individuals self-centred and insensitive to the needs of others, partly due to a loss of emotional empathy, the capacity to recognize and understand the emotions of other people. Because of the lifestyles we lead and the things we are exposed to (dangerous sports, fast cars, motorbikes, alcohol-related accidents), TBIs are becoming more common. The resulting empathy deficits can have significant negative repercussions on social functioning and quality of life. A recent study shows evidence of a relationship between physiological responses to anger and a reduction of emotional empathy post-injury. Researchers identified that those with TBI generally scored lower in emotional empathy and were less responsive, specifically to angry faces, than other people (De Sousa et al. 2011). Clearly this suggests that interventions to help build empathy post-injury need to be considered as part of the recovery and rehabilitation process.

Undoubtedly some of the responses and behaviours of people with low empathy are hard to deal with and can be particularly frustrating in the context of long-term relationships. We acknowledge that not everyone with low empathy is discussed here, but we hope we have covered enough of the issue for you to recognize if it applies to you or someone in your family. In the next chapter we explore ways people of low empathy can increase their awareness of others' feelings. We also highlight ways to improve communications and daily life when it's shared with a person who has lower than average empathy.

6

Managing relations with people of low empathy

In this chapter we continue our discussion of people with low empathy – those like moody Michaela in Chapter 1 and John with undiagnosed AS in Chapter 2. Despite their initial low empathy, people at points two to three on the empathy spectrum have better chances of moving up in position than those at point zero, though they are often restricted by what can be a pretty rigid mindset. All the same, small changes can make a big difference to the quality of everyday life.

Living made easy – or easier

Strategies for improving communication with people with autism and AS, whether or not they have a diagnosis, or even want one, include:

- Do discuss what you observe – if you think your partner, parent or child has autistic tendencies, it may be worth discussing your concerns with them and seeing if they wish to take it up with your family doctor.
- If they do not want to seek medical advice, respect their point of view. It must be the individual's decision in the end. Being open with one another about concerns and difficulties is the key to improving your communication.
- Don't make assumptions about what the other person is feeling as people with autism and AS are hard to interpret in the usual way.
- For the reason above, don't assume no eye contact is a sign that the other person is shifty or frequently lying. In people with autism and AS, poor eye contact is common.
- Many people with autism and AS *learn* non-verbal communication as opposed to spontaneously reacting and picking up the

skills from observing someone else using them. In the event of an inappropriate response (a smile, say, when you are telling them something sad), explain – without being patronizing – why there are better ways to react. Clear up any confusion they may have picked up during the course of the conversation.

- Avoid ambiguity – in particular the use of metaphor, which may be taken quite literally. Instead adopt a more direct way of communicating. Writing things down helps.

- Individuals with autism and AS can be highly sensitive to criticism because they've often experienced a lifetime of criticism and rejection. Constant criticism can lead not only to constant misunderstandings but lower self-esteem.

- Ensure that the 'rules' of conversation are adhered to – that is, that you both take turns speaking and listening as this will, over time, improve everyone's conversational skills.

- If one individual can't understand another's feelings, compromise might be the best approach – 'If we do it this way this time, next time you can have your way.'

- It can aid understanding if things are written down in a straightforward way, say in an email or letter, especially if deep feelings and complex issues are involved.

- Negotiate – people with autism and AS often find social situations exhausting but socializing is important to healthy relations, so take time to negotiate activities that individuals would like to do on their own, as well as with their friends and family.

- If your partner is autistic or has AS, as much as you are in a partnership remember to hold on to and assert your own independence.

- Have a network of friends – you need other people around who can supply you with the depth of emotional understanding and empathy you need.

- For those with difficulty socializing – those who identify themselves as having AS or entrenched behaviours associated with low empathy – there are many relevant websites and online communities and support groups that can lead the way to online friendships and actual social events.

Dealing with frustration and anger – theirs and yours!

Here are five ways to deal with unintentionally difficult people:

Step back before you respond – your natural response to a difficult person may be a critical riposte. Try not to react this way! Trust that the other person does not mean to be difficult. Take time to think of your response, instead of reacting immediately. The more you can separate the behaviour from the person, the less likely is it that you'll view their words or actions as a personal attack.

Stop wishing they were different – difficult people are not irritating on purpose. The best way to see a change in them is to change your own thinking and behaviour about them.

Approach each interaction with an open mind – really listen to what the other person has to say and remain open to his or her viewpoint. When people feel your support they will be more willing to engage with you.

Acknowledge differences in your points of view but don't argue – our first reaction might be to come out with an angry or defensive retort but this may result in the conversation escalating into an argument or the other person walking away. An effective approach is to acknowledge her or his viewpoint and suggest that there may be more than one way to deal with the issue in question. This approach positions you as equal partners and may well lead to a better solution.

Don't be a difficult person yourself! – it is easy to identify someone else being difficult, but how often do you acknowledge that you can be difficult as well, especially when you feel stressed or tired? Recognize what triggers your own responses. Take responsibility for your actions and view yourself from the other person's perspective so that you don't become the difficult person that others avoid.

Coping with specific behavioural problems

Obsessive–compulsive disorder, addiction and eating disorders are all entrenched behaviours that differ in severity. Today a vast array of literature on recovery from such behaviours exists and is readily available from bookshops and the internet. Online resources and peer groups are also available. Some of these resources are extremely useful, some less so. You will have to rely upon your powers of discrimination and your own ideas of what will work for you and your unique situation when making use of available information and support, so be discerning.

If you notice the warning signs of any of these behaviours in a friend or family member, you may be hesitant to say anything for fear of being mistaken or saying the wrong thing and alienating the person. Although it's undeniably difficult to bring up such a sensitive issue, don't let these worries keep you from voicing reasonable concerns.

People with problem behaviours are often afraid to ask for help. Some are struggling just as much as you are to find a way to start a conversation about their problem, while others have such low self-esteem they simply don't feel they deserve any help. But the problem will only get worse if it goes unacknowledged, and the emotional and other damage can be severe. The sooner you start to help your partner, daughter or son, the better the chances of recovery. When you communicate your concerns, try to:

- Focus on feelings and relationships. Share your memories of specific times when you felt concerned about the person's behaviour. Explain that you think these things may indicate that there could be a problem.

- Express concern about behaviour but do respect privacy. Your partner or child may well appreciate knowing that you are concerned and ask for help.

- Avoid power struggles over behaviour. Don't demand change; avoid scare tactics, angry outbursts and put-downs. Trying to force someone to change behaviour when that person is not ready can make things worse.

- Do whatever you can to promote self-confidence and the belief that pulling off enduring change is indeed possible.

- Avoid prescribing both the speed of change and the solution. The pace of change and the solution must be determined by the individual.

- Don't become so preoccupied with the other person's problems that you neglect your own needs. Make sure you have your own support so that you can provide it in turn.

- Recovering from any entrenched behaviour problem takes time. There are no quick solutions or miracle cures so it's important to have patience and compassion.

Tips on better communication

Effective communication helps us better understand a person or situation and enables us to resolve differences, build trust and an environment where problem-solving, affection and caring can flourish. Effective communication also requires you to understand the emotion behind the words and actions of another person. Listening and observational skills are two of the most important aspects of effective communication. Successful listening means understanding not just the words being communicated but also how speakers feel about what they're communicating.

Developing the ability to understand and use non-verbal communication can also help you connect with others, express what you really mean, navigate challenging situations and build better relationships at home and work. In the case of observing people with low empathy, this means becoming more aware of their differences and their gestures of communication. It also means not judging them unfairly or comparing their actions and responses unfavourably with your own. Good communication sometimes entails looking for humour in the situation – humour can be a great way to relieve stress when communicating. And be willing to compromise – sometimes, if you can both bend a little, you'll be able to find a happy middle ground. If you realize that the other person cares much more about something than you do, compromise may be easier for you. Finally, sometimes it is necessary to agree to disagree – take a quick break and move away from the situation.

Table 1 outlines the different stances people commonly adopt. This is adapted from one of the bestselling self-help books ever published, Thomas A. Harris's *I'm OK – You're OK*, first published in 1967 but still in print and highly relevant today. Ours is an abridged version of Harris's identified life positions. Harris had a fourth position, 'I'm not OK, you're not OK', which can arise in children and adults who have been abused, but is far less common. The position in the middle – the 'I'm OK, you're OK' status – is your best bet and the place to aim for.

Table 1 Who's OK?

You're OK, I'm not	I'm OK, you're OK	I'm OK, you're not
Belief	**Belief**	**Belief**
Your view is more important than mine, so it doesn't matter what I think.	I believe and act as if we both deserve respect. We're equally entitled to have things done our way.	I believe I'm entitled to have things done my way, because I'm right. You're wrong and not entitled to do things your way.
Consequences	**Consequences**	**Consequences**
These people give in to others, don't get what they want or need, and have self-critical thoughts.	These people generally have good relationships, are happy to compromise but don't disregard their own wants and needs.	These people often upset others and themselves, and often feel angry and resentful.

Emotional awareness helps you understand yourself and other people, so become acquainted with your emotions – all of them. They are not good or bad, just messengers trying to tell you something. Many people ignore or conceal from themselves strong emotions like anger, sadness and fear, yet our ability to communicate effectively depends on being connected to these feelings. If you insist on communicating only on a rational level, it will impair your ability to understand others fully, resolve conflicts or build a meaningful connection with them.

If you are more clued in to your feelings they will be more likely to come and go. You don't have to choose between feeling and thinking – you can feel as you think, think as you feel. Emotional awareness or 'mindfulness', as it is often called, is a skill that most people can learn. Mindfulness exercises are freely available on the internet (see Useful addresses).

Available support

If a family member or friend has what seems to you to be a specific behavioural problem, voicing your concerns directly and inviting discussion of them is an important first step. Talking to your doctor or contacting a helping organization is the likely next step. Sources of support include the following (and see also Useful addresses):

Therapy/counselling

Individual and group therapy can help the individual explore the issues underlying the behaviour problem, improve self-esteem and learn healthy ways of responding to stress and emotional pain. Family therapy is also effective for dealing with the impact of the problem on the entire family.

In the case of eating disorders, nutritional counsellors are often involved in the treatment. They can help to set dietary goals, and the individual to achieve a healthy weight.

Support groups

For the past few decades, researchers have been evaluating the effects of self-help and mutual aid groups. Most research studies of self-help groups have found important benefits of participation. Attending a support group can help an individual struggling with a specific behavioural problem to feel less alone and ashamed. Run by peers rather than professionals, support groups provide a safe environment to share experiences, advice, encouragement and coping strategies.

Treatment

Outpatient, hospital-based or residential care may be required when there are severe physical outcomes from enduring behavioural problems, as may be the case with eating disorders or chronic and excessive alcohol and drug use. Moreover acute withdrawal symptoms are sometimes experienced when an individual abruptly stops drinking or drug-taking, a situation that can sometimes necessitate medical treatment and close monitoring.

To try out: a self-compassion exercise for carers and family members

The first step towards changing the way you treat and respond to others is to treat yourself well and be less self-critical. It may be that you are so often self-critical that you don't even notice that you are. Many of us need a little encouragement to think better of ourselves on the road to greater self-compassion.

1 Become more aware of how often you engage in self-critical thinking. Whenever you're feeling bad about something, try immediately to capture what you've just said to yourself. What words do you actually use when you're self-critical? It might be useful to write them down.

2 Make an active effort to soften that self-critical inner voice, but do so with compassion rather than self-judgement. Reframe the observations made by your inner critic in a friendly, positive way. If you're having trouble thinking of what words to use, you might want to imagine what a very compassionate friend would say to you in this situation. Again, it might help to write the words down.

In the next chapter our attention turns to people with middling levels of empathy and the problem of apathy in families.

7

The in-betweeners

Do you have a family member like Andy, the single parent we met in Chapter 2, who seems indifferent to your concerns? Someone who doesn't want to get involved or respond to the concerns of one of your children who is being bullied at school? Does your family member sit on the fence during an argument, imagining this is fair minded when in reality it means a family problem goes unaddressed – for example, refusing to express a view about whether or not it is acceptable for your teenage daughter to stay out all night? Does your sibling refuse to discuss the long-term care of a sick and elderly parent? Does your spouse not come to your aid when you're intimidated by your overbearing father-in-law? Or what if you are the one who responds impassively to certain situations?

Family members who show so little interest in the affairs of others could almost be called neglectful. In this chapter we introduce the **in-betweeners**, those whose default position is the middle of the empathy spectrum, which is the point on it where the majority of us lie. On the whole the midpoint of the spectrum is a favourable place to be, where neither too little nor too much empathy is experienced. But in-betweeners may still have some difficulties expressing empathy. In this chapter we put forward the idea that apathy is a state of mind that has a deterrent effect and blocks empathy. Apathy often is a defence mechanism that silences empathy, takes away the problem of deciding which way to turn, and renders us pretty useless and inactive companions. In this chapter we spell out our individual and collective need to cast aside apathy and indifference.

Empathy and apathy

By definition empathy is the opposite of apathy. Empathy is the ability to understand and share the feelings of another, whereas apathy is a lack of interest, enthusiasm or concern. Some believe that both empathy and apathy are contagious in that they spread from one person to another. Thus one person who acts with empathy or apathy potentially has the power to infect or influence everyone around them.

There are some emotional states that should not be confused with apathy, such as emotional flatness (being unable to express emotions). In such cases individuals often show little or no emotional expressiveness, and may show no signs of emotion as most of us know and experience it. They may speak in a monotonous voice and lack facial expressions, and/or appear extremely uninterested in things around them. In some cultures emotional flatness is viewed as mental disorder (associated with schizophrenia, for example), while in others displaying little emotion is considered a positive trait, a way of presenting one's self in the customary fashion. One way, perhaps, to view the difference between emotional flatness and apathy is to regard the latter as a way of reacting, or rather not reacting, to a given situation.

As we suggested earlier, apathy can result when people find themselves between 'a rock and a hard place' – in a difficult situation and not knowing which way to turn. In certain circumstances, especially when confronted with a tricky situation, we can be rendered impassive.

Apathy can immobilize us when we feel the impulse to compete and cooperate at the same time. Cooperation can be subdivided into friendly cooperation and hostile cooperation – though both have an element of competition. An example of **friendly cooperation** is the coming together of people to compete against other individuals or groups, say in a football team. **Hostile cooperation** is cooperation that exists between competitors. For example, athletes cooperate with one another and abide by the event's rules, not for mutual benefit but to prevent their being disqualified from the competition. In an event like sprinting it is in the individual athlete's interests to adhere to the rules in order to compete and have a chance of winning. In this way competitors cooperate because the rewards prove greater when they do.

But suppose one of the sprinters gets ahead because the official judging the event is indifferent to the situation and his stagnant view obscures the sprinter's false start. We touched on this sort of behaviour in Chapter 3 in discussing the sociopathic transaction, where apathetic and indifferent individuals are engaged passively or otherwise take part in the manipulator's sport.

We call people who connive in hostile competition in this passive way **apaths**. Their apathy is often only a temporary affliction and they may only behave this way in the heat of the moment and later come to regret it. The reasons people join forces with aggressive competitive types are manifold: they may fear punishment or maltreatment if they don't go along with them; may bear a grudge towards the targeted individual, team or social group or feel anger towards them, or have no real connection with them; may go along with the situation purely out of boredom! Apathy can thus be less calculated than we have so far described it. It can simply be the first reaction to perceived danger and an avoidance strategy engaged in in the hope that the problem will go away.

Whether calculated or relatively ingenuous, apaths end up walking in and out of situations in a trance-like state, as if their consciences have fallen asleep. In this state apathy becomes not simply a lack of empathy but is a betrayal of it. It allows us to turn a collective blind eye to abuses, crimes and barbarities. We ignore humans who are suffering because at that moment we don't view them as our equals, rather as others, objects and 'its'.

We have described apathetic behaviour and apaths as analogous with the townsfolk in the Hans Christian Andersen tale, 'The Emperor's New Clothes', who 'see' the Emperor wearing new clothes when in fact he is naked. Apathy at the level of the community represents fear, collective denial and social hypocrisy, and at its worst takes the form of collusion. In our case study of an in-betweener from Chapter 2 (see pp. 20–1), Andy refuses to find out what is the matter with his daughter, or express his concerns that she may be developing an eating disorder, because he fears the consequences of taking action. To be unresponsive like Andy in this way can result from **learned helplessness**.

Learned helplessness, which we noted at the end of Chapter 4, is when someone has learned over time to behave helplessly and fails to respond even though there are opportunities to help themselves and possibly other people too. Andy probably behaved as he did because he likely couldn't bear hearing how his daughter really feels about herself and may have had concerns about it affecting their relationship. For all we know Andy may have learned from past experience that talking about personal fears and problems only gets him into trouble, so he avoids doing so. Perhaps Andy had problems of a not too different sort as a teenager but never told anyone for fear of rejection. Whatever the reason, Andy has learned that inaction feels safer than confronting the issue head on.

Learned helplessness is not unique to humans – take the extreme case of ants. Ants communicate information by leaving pheromone tracks. A moving ant leaves a quantity of pheromone on the ground to mark its way and an individual ant encountering a trail made by other ants will follow it. On the rare occasion that a group of army ants are separated from the main foraging party after losing the pheromone track, they begin to follow one another, forming a continuously rotating circle, and eventually die of exhaustion. This behaviour is called the 'ant mill', otherwise known as the 'ant circle of death'.

This shows us how apathy and collective follow-my-leader behaviour can be detrimental to ourselves and others. It is tempting to look at apathy as merely a problem of the individual but it is not. It is a problem of global proportions and incredibly hazardous. Apathy is one of those traits that can damage people and political systems.

The problem was demonstrated effectively in the 1960s when Stanley Milgram, a professor at Yale University, set up an experiment to test the human propensity to obey orders. A participant was asked to take the role of 'teacher' and to administer an electric shock to the 'learner' whenever the learner answered a question incorrectly. The experiment was stopped after the subject supposedly had been given the maximum 450-volt shock three times in succession (in fact the learners did not receive a shock and were faking their physical response). As many as 62.5 per cent of the 'teachers' administered the final massive 450-volt shock, though many were very uncomfortable doing so. Milgram's experiment, despite the ethical issues it raises, has been repeated many times over and yielded consistent results. What it suggests is that a person of authority can strongly influence other people's behaviour, which renders it a useful phenomenon in that it makes it easy for an authority/government to establish order and control, but in the wrong hands has such power and influence that it can have appalling consequences.

Apathy in adulthood and in relationships

As we emotionally mature through childhood and into adulthood, we learn and take on board moral standards that we absorb from the individuals around us – from society at large and the people who make up the community we live in. All being well, the development of these moral standards passes through several stages in childhood and adolescence, moving from avoidance of punishment to avoidance of disapproval and rejection and finally to avoidance of guilt and self-recrimination. With apathy we dodge the last step in the process.

The more a person avoids dealing with their own problems, needs and wants, the more their relationships with others are adversely affected. People experience apathy when they lose hope in getting what they want or need. Apathy sometimes precedes depression, which occurs after this loss of hope. What often starts as a niggling concern and a feeling that 'something isn't right' turns into a sense of hopelessness if not addressed. While hopelessness is not in itself apathy, it can soon turn that way when it forms into indifference. Avoiding dealing with our concerns in our relationships in the long term can have a terminal effect on them. That said, taking the wrong kind of action – for instance, repeatedly criticizing your partner, siblings or friends – is likely to discourage them rather than encourage them to take affirmative action, and give them the message that they aren't 'good enough'. Eventually they may come to the conclusion that whatever they do is never good enough and give up hope and stop trying. Everyone is responsible for their own actions, but our own actions can strongly influence other people to choose apathy or some other negative attitudes and actions. A relationship is two people interacting. We must take responsibility for our own role in our relationships and how we influence the reactions of others. Healing and progress in our relationships can be delayed though avoidance, so the only real remedy is to do some positive work, such as the sorts of activities suggested in Chapter 8.

Apathy versus ambivalence

Whether you express empathy in particular circumstances depends on what you are empathic about and how easy it is for you to feel certain things in your own mind. Sometimes we can be uncertain about how we feel about situations in which we find ourselves, and become immobilized by our confusion. This is called being in a state of **ambivalence**. Apathy and ambivalence are often used interchangeably but there are some differences. When we are apathetic about something we usually don't wish to share or expose a view of the person or issue involved. Someone in an apathetic state will appear indecisive and unemotional. By contrast someone in a state of ambivalence is in an emotional state and in a sort of stalemate between opposing thoughts and feelings. A person in this state can want and not want something at the same time, hence experiencing an emotionally laden and frustrating tug of war, which results in an inability to make a decision.

In many cases ambivalence involves being caught in a conflict of values. Someone stuck in ambivalence is not necessarily being irrational – they can be perfectly rational in weighing up opposing views. It makes perfect sense that someone facing an important life decision or choice would struggle to determine which course to take and feel unwilling to go forward until the right course seems clear. People have the capacity to consider alternatives, imagine different perspectives and futures and act so as to choose one direction as opposed to another – and yet because our perspective is always limited we can never be certain that the choice we make will bring the results we hope for. It is apprehension and uncertainty that causes the stagnant state of ambivalence.

Ambivalence can render a person immobile in much the same way as someone experiencing apathy. Ambivalence is a perfectly normal human response and we experience it on a daily basis, whether we arrive in that state cogitating over what to have for dinner or deliberating over some truly life-changing course of action. It is usually only when deciding the serious – life-changing – stuff that ambivalence overwhelms us. Having to make decisions under conditions of uncertainty means we frequently oscillate between thinking about our dilemma and, finding ourselves wanting to go in two directions at the same time, putting that dilemma out of mind, thus going over and over it.

The good news among the concerns we raise here about middling levels of empathy is that in-betweeners usually are only temporarily afflicted with ambivalence and apathy. In Chapter 8 we consider ways in-betweeners might become better connected to their feelings and freer in expressing their emotions, and thus able to enjoy more of a sense of connectedness with other people.

8

Resolving apathy

All his anxiety resolved itself into a sigh and dissolved into apathy and drowsiness.

Ivan Goncharov, *Oblomov* (1859)

In this chapter we explore the problem of apathy and what those periodically afflicted with it can do to avoid being impassive to family events and situations. Goncharov's novel *Oblomov* was written over a century and a half ago and highlights the perennial nature of the problem. Oblomov was a man so lazy that he gave up his job and found himself in debt. He was too apathetic to do anything about his problems so he delayed change and ended up risking losing the love of his life.

So if you, your partner or even your elderly parent are prone to apathy and have an annoying tendency to sit on the fence in relation to family affairs, one way to limit the effects is to increase awareness of your feelings and the feelings of others around you. The key to ridding oneself of apathy is to avoid becoming too practised in self-trickery and more practised in recognizing your own and others' feelings. Here we talk about recognizing and unleashing emotions in order to express empathy more freely.

Know your own mind

Empathy builds on self-awareness: the more open we are to our own emotions, the more skilled we are in reading and concerning ourselves with our own feelings and the feelings of others. Or put another way, the less we dissociate from our own feelings the less likely we are to dissociate from the feelings and concerns of others. The aim of this chapter is to help you find ways and the inner resources to respond with enriched emotional articulacy. At the end of the chapter we include some self-compassion and empathy exercises for you to try.

Some people are fantastically empathic when it comes to caring but have very little empathy at all when it comes to dealing with someone else's outrage or anger. It is not uncommon for people to sidestep certain feelings and avoid expressing emotions that they are uncomfortable with. Some close down in the face of violence and abuse, and cut off completely from emotions they are frightened of in themselves. In this section we explore ways in which you can harness your emotions instead of avoiding them.

Making the most of your emotional intelligence

The psychologist Daniel Goleman suggests that all emotions are impulses to act. Needed for coping and surviving, the emotions of fear, anger, happiness, love, surprise, disgust and sadness send signals to the brain that release hormones to give strength to the necessary reactions (Goleman 1998). Being alert to our feelings is important to thought and vice versa, and emotional thought leads to action. This situation suggests that humans are of two minds: the **emotional mind** and the **rational mind**. One mind feels and the other thinks. In the emotional mind lodge impulsive, powerful and often illogical feelings, while the rational mind affords us the ability to think and reflect. Emotion informs the rational mind, which moderates the involvement and expression of our emotions.

Being able to pick up on our own distress helps us recognize another person's distress and respond in appropriate and supportive ways. Being alert to our own and others' emotional states requires emotional intelligence. **Emotional intelligence** means we have acquired a good balance between our rational and emotional minds. This is important in the elimination of both apathy and ambivalence, and where emotional and rational minds are caught in a struggle. Psychologists define emotional intelligence as the ability to reason with emotion. Goleman, a major contributor in this area, divides emotional intelligence into five main areas (Goleman 1995):

Knowing your emotions – recognizing a feeling as it happens gives you greater certainty about your feelings and helps you make personal decisions.

Managing emotions – the ability to handle feelings builds on self-awareness. Those who excel in managing their emotions are more likely to bounce back quickly from setbacks and upsets.

Motivating yourself – people who can channel their emotions towards a goal can motivate themselves to achieve their goals.

Recognizing emotions in others – people who demonstrate empathy are more attuned to what others may need or want.

Handling relationships – the skill of dealing with other people's emotions is the basis of the art of relationships.

In order to enhance our interpersonal abilities we need to establish our own distinctive style for handling our feelings. John Mayer and Alexander Stevens suggest these styles for dealing with emotions (Mayer and Stevens 1994):

Self-aware – these people are aware of their moods, are sure of their boundaries and have a positive outlook on life. They manage their emotions and do not ruminate over bad moods.

Engulfed – these people are consumed by their emotions, feel helpless to escape them, are not aware of their feelings and therefore lose perspective. The result is that they feel they have little control over their emotions.

Accepting – these people tend to accept their different moods and don't necessarily try to change them.

Thinking out loud

We need to become more clued up about what we feel and think by listening to our internal dialogue – our thoughts and feelings. If you have trouble listening to your inner self when you feel overwhelmed or emotionally fatigued, a preliminary step is listening to yourself think out loud.

To do this, find somewhere where you are able to relax and are unlikely to be disturbed, away from other members of the family. Then listen to both sides, or as the communication expert Elayne Savage puts it, 'your voice of confidence and your voice of doubt' (Savage 2002). If you only listen to one voice you are, in effect, rejecting the other. If listening in this way seems an unnatural thing to do at first, instead try writing a 'What I have to gain' and a 'What I have to lose' list.

You might discover you have conflicting thoughts that you struggle to reconcile. This is called being ambivalent or in a state of 'two minds'. Often in such cases, allowing yourself time to ponder and weigh up your concerns and choices is really valuable. The process of reflecting on your thoughts and feelings in this way is often all that is needed to unleash you from that stuck state. But if ambivalence immobilizes you and you are gripped by fear, what then? You can help yourself move forward by naming the fear. So ask yourself, 'What is my fear?' Try to describe it. Is it fear of rejection, of failure, of success? Or do you fear being judged or punished? Naming the fear out loud and writing it down can sometimes help. Try it – see if it allows you to view things differently and recognize the route out of your state of 'stuckness'. Ambivalence, like apathy, can render us inactive. Although our feelings, thoughts, behaviours, traits, deficits and strengths can't possibly be fully transparent, at least by being more self-examining we become conscious of how we feel about everyday concerns and issues.

Don't let fear hem you in

Sometimes we fear moving forward, not because we haven't made our minds up about our options but because we fear change itself. For most of us, preserving the status quo matters most. We fear change because with change there is often loss, and with loss there is often sadness and grief. Sometimes we fear so much what we might lose with change that the fear immobilizes us and keeps us stuck. We find that we don't know which way to turn or how to act. But with grief and loss there can be space for creative engagement, participation, care and concern. When it's time to face your concerns, find somewhere quiet where you can go into contemplative mode and take heed of what's on your mind:

- Approach any fear or anxiety you have with detachment. Become more aware of it by noticing *what* you are afraid of or anxious about, *when* you feel like this and *where* you feel it in your body.
- In your mind's eye, really look at this fear or anxiety. How big or small is it? Do you need to confront it – or is there a way of manoeuvring around it?

Ambivalence-busting strategies

Once you have got more in touch with your fears and concerns, the next step is to neutralize it. The following statements and questions to ask yourself are intended to help you dislodge your fear.

- Recognize that ambivalence is part of everyday life.
- Remember that part of the clarification process is to find out what it is you are struggling with.

So try answering the following questions:

- Do I really want to continue down this path? I could retrace my steps and go down a different path.
- If I choose to carry on on this path and act on the issues facing me, what is likely to happen?
- What would it mean if I failed to act?
- What are the paybacks to me and others if I take action?

Conquering fear

If fear is still getting in the way, it may be that you need to reframe your thinking. Keep these statements handy for times when you really need to conquer that fear:

1 Value courage – don't cling to things just for security.
2 Appreciate the difference between being fearful and being cautious.
3 View fear as a call to arms – a signal to take action.
4 Reframe fear as excitement.

Distress reaction

There are times when our lack of response to others comes not from being in two minds but from the shock of witnessing appalling acts or events. This is called **trauma-induced apathy**. Distressing events such as sudden illness, an unexpected death in the family, abuse and accidents can be traumatic, and responding requires great physical and mental energy. Once the worst is over, people involved usually feel exhausted and emotional. Distress reactions after such events can occur hours, days, weeks or even months later.

Afterwards you may find yourself trying to make sense of what has happened and how and why it happened – why you were involved, why you feel the way you do, whether the experience has changed your view on life and so on.

Suggestions to help sort things out in your mind include talking over your thoughts and feelings with trusted friends and loved ones. However, if you don't feel like talking there are other things you can do, such as:

- Keep a journal of your thoughts and feelings;
- Keep to your normal routine;
- Keep yourself occupied with social events, hobbies or favoured activities;
- Set aside time to relax.

The distress reaction is a normal response to abnormal and harrowing situations. Most people recover and feel normal again in time and normality can resume fairly swiftly with adequate support. However, some people may find themselves 'stuck'. A prolonged distress reaction can cause other problems, such as relationship difficulties. For instance, if you get low and depressed you may withdraw from other people's company. Without help to move on the reaction may become a way of life. Counselling or therapy could prove helpful – see Useful addresses for internet resources with information about different kinds.

As highlighted in Chapter 7, prolonged or chronic apathy is associated with such medical conditions as depression, Alzheimer's disease, schizophrenia, bipolar disorder and Asperger syndrome, to name a few. Some medications and the heavy use of drugs may bring apathy as a side effect. However, doctors do not explicitly deal with apathy or view it as a condition that requires a medical response. It is probably best not to over-medicalize everyday sorts of problems such as this anyway, so don't be afraid to try to combat apathy in yourself. Tell yourself you can free yourself from it if you find the right approach. Your best bet is to have people around you for stimulation – family and friends. If you are short of friends then get outside and mingle – going and sitting in a café is a good start. Go on – immerse yourself in the social whirl!

From apathy to action

Apathy can be an obstacle to living life fully. It keeps us from forming alliances and feeling connections to our fellow human beings. Apathy tends to be a lonely state, one that keeps us from doing what we can to help others and that, in turn, keeps us from asking others for help. Here are our five top tips for dealing with and overcoming apathy:

Connect with others who value empathy – we need the support and encouragement of others who value empathy and want to transform society, so go out and find like-minded people. There are plenty there – you just need to go and find them!

Be mindful and alert to apathy in yourself and others – avoid other apaths whenever and wherever possible. Be alert to what others say and don't say, what they do and don't do. Ignore apathetic comments like, 'Nobody else minds, so why should I?', 'Lighten up' or 'Who cares anyway?'. Act on things you are impassioned about and issues that are important to you.

Practise self-compassion – this means being mindful to care and value yourself. Also showing yourself small kindnesses each day should help you express empathy for others more readily (we provide some ideas and exercises to try in the next section, Building self-compassion).

Lead by example – those who are not completely infected with apathy may be energized into action and follow your lead.

Don't wait for the prisoners, they can free themselves! – once you've opened the door to opportunity, don't hang about to free other apathetic people – they may complain or even try to block your actions. Reframe your thoughts and feel happy that your bit of good in the world may have benefited others also, rather than wait for them to see things as you do.

Building self-compassion

In her book *The Gifts of Imperfection*, the researcher Brené Brown advises us to let go of anxieties about our imperfections. She says we should stop being concerned by what others think and be sufficiently at ease with ourselves to say, 'I am enough'. Self-compassion means letting go of concern about how other people view us. It is about letting go of the idea of being perfect, allowing ourselves to feel and express emotion more freely, letting go of fear, learning to trust our intuition (gut feelings), not comparing ourselves with others and having to be in control. Self-compassion grows from accepting our imperfections, being creative and allowing ourselves some fun! When people are confused about their own feelings they often have difficulty recognizing the feelings of others.

In reality, though people often say they want to be more self-compassionate they usually don't and continue to be self-critical, so that when a problem arises they have difficulties. In order to practise self-compassion we need to:

1 Be mindful – recognize and acknowledge when we are in distress.
2 Acknowledge that suffering is a shared experience and part of life. We might also acknowledge that whatever suffering or distress we're experiencing, others are likely to relate to it.
3 Be kind to ourselves and acknowledge that our desire is to be free from suffering or distress, whether or not we see that we have somehow contributed to it.

Learning to be self-compassionate is a skill – it might take a while before you feel good at it. Being self-compassionate instead of self-critical offers you a powerful tool for coping in daily life. To get you started, here are some situations where you might try applying some self-compassion:

- When you're trying hard but not being as effective as you would like.
- When you compare yourself unfavourably to someone else.
- When you make a mistake.
- When you feel guilt or shame.
- When perfection isn't attainable.
- When you perceive a flaw in yourself.
- When you're having a recurring problem and feel overwhelmed by it.
- When you are in two minds or ambivalent.
- When you feel angry, jealous or selfish and criticize yourself for having those feelings.

- When anxiety or other emotions are making it hard to respond as you would wish to.
- When you're experiencing regret about a decision you made.
- When you want to do the right thing but are concerned that it's too late.

Empathy building

Exercise 1

At home and whenever you are engaged in a one-to-one and private conversation with a family member:

Listen to and watch the talker – when the talker is speaking, maintain good eye contact. Hear the talker's words and tone of voice. Observe her or his facial expression and other non-verbal messages. From what you see and hear, look for suggestions of feelings.

Listen to your own gut reactions – mentally put yourself in the talker's situation. Imagine what you would do and how you would be feeling. If you have had experiences similar to the talker's, then recall and mentally recreate the feelings you had. The talker may be feeling the same way you did in the same situation.

Utilize your memory – you will have a general idea about how someone in a similar situation to the talker would respond in the same or similar circumstances. You may have known others who have had the same issues as the talker, so try to recall how they said they felt and how they acted.

Have faith in the talker and his or her ability to sort things out – when you listen empathically you provide an opportunity to make the talker feel comfortable enough to explore his or her situation and feelings. Your role is not to make decisions for the talker. Remember that ambivalence is entirely natural – it's a mechanism we benefit from being alert to because it forces us to stop and reflect on our everyday concerns and dilemmas. Listening to others discuss their concerns when they are in a state of ambivalence can help them to make decisions and move them to take action.

Exercise 2

For families and people living together to identify personal and shared morals and values:

Work out morals and values individually and collectively – this will help you understand where everyone is coming from. It will also test your abilities to listen, communicate and cooperate with one another. If some common ground is identified, see if you can incorporate these values into everyday family life.

Empathy is central to establishing strong relationships. It is at the heart of effective communication. It fuels understanding and forgiveness, and bonds us together – essential traits in strong and successful relationships. In the next chapter we highlight empaths and superempaths and the pros and cons of being a highly empathic person in an indifferent society.

9

Super empathy and problems of the highly perceptive

This chapter discusses the problems sometimes faced by highly empathic individuals like Barry, the exceptionally kind and loving grandfather who featured in a case study in Chapter 2 (pp. 23–4). Barry is one of those perceptive and sensitive people who pick up on unspoken issues and shoulder other people's emotions. Perhaps you have a family member who tends to shoulder other people's problems; or your partner suffers from social anxiety and won't go out much; or you are the one who shoulders everyone's problems and don't have enough time or space to deal with your own.

Highly empathic individuals, otherwise known as superempaths, represent the pinnacle of what it is to be human and humane. All the same, living with such sensitive individuals can be difficult. Many of the problems superempaths encounter are due to the fact that they live in a culture of indifference. Pushed to the extreme, they can feel so overwhelmed by the indifference of others that they isolate themselves to cope. Empathy expressed by someone with sufficient self-compassion means that a balanced state in that person's everyday relations and communications can be achieved – that is, the 'I'm OK, you're OK' status (see Table 1 in Chapter 6, p. 68). But having too much empathy and too little self-compassion can tip us off beam and into the 'You're OK, I'm not' position, just as it did in Barry's case.

The talents of the superempath

It is important to notice that empaths are everywhere, in every culture throughout the world, but because they don't tend to make 'a song and dance' of their talents you have to know what you are looking for.

Empathy has an emotional component (feelings that provide

us with the capacity to respond with an appropriate emotion to another's mental states) and a cognitive element (the capacity to understand another's perspective or mental state). The emotional component could be subdivided into empathic concern (the inclination to experience feelings of sympathy and compassion towards others in response to their suffering) and empathic distress (the inclination to experience self-centred feelings of discomfort and anxiety in response to another's suffering). Highly empathic people tend to experience high levels of these elements, though one constituent may take precedence over another. Some are more easily brought to tears over seeing another person in distress, while others might experience a great deal of empathic anger (a form of empathic distress). Indeed, they may feel compelled to act if they witness some atrocity or monstrous act. Empathic anger, if acted upon, is anger that is prosocial in form, for it serves as a vehicle to protect the group and its members and is an act of assistance and cooperation. Empathic anger is the driving force of many activists and social reformers.

Empaths experience compassion towards family, children, friends, complete strangers, pets, plants and inanimate objects. In a sense, empaths are the complete communication package. They possess the ability to sense others on many different levels, observing what another is saying, feeling and thinking, and they can become very proficient at reading other people's body language; though this is not in itself empathy, it is an advantage that comes from being observant of others.

Being highly empathic often means being highly sensitive too. Highly sensitive is a term commonly used in describing one's ability to sense or detect another's emotions and feelings, and is used interchangeably with the term empath. One of the most obvious empathic bonds is that between parent and child. Mothers show recognizable signs of empathy in the early days of conception, and this rapidly increases after birth. Children will mirror the feelings and thoughts of their parents and siblings because they are in tune with them and around them on a daily basis. It is wonderful to grow up with empathic parents because these fortunate children are less likely to suppress their abilities and more likely to accept their natural talents.

In general, empaths tend to be peacemakers and can be loyal

friends, though they are just as easily crushed if the friendship is abused. If they have been mistreated by others, over time they may become far more wary and selective. They are good listeners and complete strangers find it easy to talk to them, even about personal things. Added to this, empaths are often quiet achievers. They can find it hard to take a compliment for they're more inclined to point out another's positive attributes. Nevertheless they are highly expressive, often insightful and willing to talk openly.

Constricted by a culture of apathy

About one in five of us are born with heightened sensitivity to our surroundings, men and women in equal number. Being highly responsive is most likely inherited, and a large body of research suggests that the trait is innate (Aron et al. 2012). In her book *The Highly Sensitive Person* (1996), the psychologist Elaine Aron estimates that around 20 per cent of individuals have the characteristic. Aron claims that the brains of highly sensitive people have more activity and blood flow in the right hemisphere, indicating an internal rather than external view on life. Experiences that moderately affect most people can overwhelm highly sensitive people owing to their biological makeup. Highly sensitive empaths often have decreased levels of serotonin, a hormone involved in the regulation of mood, appetite and sleep and also in memory and learning. It is thought that decreased serotonin levels result from the repeated or chronic overstimulation of certain areas of the brain.

Researchers have come up with a plausible explanation for the sense of feeling overwhelmed that is often experienced by super-empaths or the highly sensitive. Aron refers to the mechanism as the **brain's two systems**. She argues that the balance of these two systems causes heightened sensitivity. One brain system is called the **behavioural activation system**. This is wired up to the parts of the brain that send messages from our senses to make our limbs move and become active. The system was probably meant to keep us searching for food and other necessities for survival. The other brain system is usually referred to as the **behavioural inhibition system**. This system is thought to make us more attentive to danger and direct us away from dangerous situations. In most of us there is a constant power struggle between these two systems, and in some people one system or other may be out of balance. For super-empaths and highly sensitive types, one of the two brain systems may win out – either they seek a quiet life away from excitement and danger, or the two brain systems remain in constant conflict, resulting in individuals seeking new things out but being conscious that they'll thus most likely end up exhausted and emotionally spent.

The ideas outlined above are derived from investigations into shyness in children by the American psychologist Jerome Kagan (Kagan 1998; Moehler et al. 2008). Kagan suggests that our dispositions are influenced to some extent by the amygdalae (Greek for 'almond', in reference to their shape), a set of neurons located deep in the brain's medial temporal lobe. We have two amygdalae, one in each brain hemisphere. The amygdalae seem to be genetically wired for a higher level of fear in some individuals. They respond to severe traumas with a lasting fear response, known as post-traumatic stress disorder or PTSD. The amygdalae receive all sorts of sensory input about sights, sounds, tastes and so on, and communicate this information to other parts of the brain involved in thought, emotional reactions and behaviour. It is thought that the amygdalae are involved in the struggle of the two brain systems because they are also in the part of the brain involved in the fight or flight response. When a person becomes frightened, the amygdalae alert another area of the brain, the hypothalamus, which in turn triggers the release of cortisol, also known as the 'stress hormone'. Kagan theorizes that some of us are born with amygdalae that are highly reactive, triggering a stress reaction in response to even a moderate stimulus. He also suggests that since these traits appear early they are likely influenced in part by our genetic makeup. Elaine Aron's research also points to genetic involvement in heightened sensitivity.

However, we humans vary in many ways – we are a lot more than the sum of our genes and biological systems. The medical research outlined above, like the culture we live in, reflects only one view of the issue, and that is one that sees empaths as defective somehow, in need of remedy. The modern view of highly empathic people as sensitive, feeble and weak needs challenging. The rest of us require these people to become emboldened and willing to educate the rest of us to act in benevolent ways.

Are you highly empathic?

Consider the following questions:

- Do other people's moods affect your mood?
- Do you pick up on other people's physical and emotional pain?
- Do you tune into and note other people's feelings easily?
- Do you experience overwhelming feelings when confronted with lots of other people and when you're in crowded places?
- Do you feel compelled to help others in physical or emotional distress?
- Do people, including strangers, often pour out their hearts to you?
- Are distressing news stories and films too distressing to look at or listen to?
- Do you care more about other people's feelings and well-being than your own?

If you responded in the affirmative to most if not all the above, the chances are you are an empath of the highest rank. This is not a scientific test – in fact very little research has been conducted in this area. All the same, if you identify with most of these statements then you are probably highly empathic. Empaths, more so superempaths, are often quiet and reflective types, who find it hard to handle a compliment. They are far more likely to point out another's positive attributes than their own. Often they are highly expressive, talk openly about themselves and have few problems talking about their feelings. Highly empathic people listen hard in order to grasp the emotional state and needs of others. They also make themselves vulnerable, removing their masks and revealing their feelings to others in order to create a strong empathic bond.

In many situations, having a strong awareness of our surroundings is beneficial because it alerts us to danger, but a tendency towards hyperawareness can become a problem if the individual becomes overstimulated and distressed. Sometimes empaths use food, alcohol or drugs to avoid or blunt the effects of feeling overcome, or in extreme circumstances may become reclusive. This extreme behaviour, usually in response to stress, is similar to narcissistic behaviour – that is, it is self-serving in nature.

Reclusive behaviour has long been associated with those in emotional pain. It is effectively illustrated in the Oscar Wilde tale, 'The Selfish Giant'. The tale, written in the late nineteenth century but still pertinent today, is a story of a selfish giant who builds a wall around his beautiful garden to keep children out. We don't know about the giant's past but the story hints at someone in emotional pain and reveals that it was always winter in the garden because no other season would visit there. Then one morning a special child brought spring back, and the giant's heart melted along with the snow. The central theme of this parable is selfishness versus selflessness.

A wrong sense of being flawed

Empaths may be gifted with high emotional intelligence and be the most intuitive and perceptive of everyone on the empathy spectrum, but their behaviour nevertheless is more often than not regarded as problematic, their natures viewed as fragile and oversensitive. All too often their talents are discounted as weakness. In a world awash with the indifferent, the highly empathic are regarded – incorrectly – as defective and flawed.

One reason for this false perception is that empaths often attract the suffering of others or suffer on their behalf. In other words they put other people's needs before their own and so end up in a situation of 'You're OK, I'm not' – see Table 2.

Once again, let us consider Barry, the kindly 80-year-old empath from Chapter 2. He finds it hard to put his needs first and think about himself. Alone after his beloved wife Eileen's dies, he avoids

Table 2 You're OK, I'm not

You're OK, I'm not
Belief
Your view is more important than mine, so it doesn't matter what I think.

other people, even his adult daughters when they have offered to help, in order to deal with his grief. As is usual in cases of 'You're OK, I'm not', Barry holds the belief that his thoughts and feelings are unimportant compared to other people. He is the sort to show concern for others, not be the one to seek comfort from them. This means he is unlikely to get what he needs, which becomes problematic for him when he is grieving and in need of emotional support. Having no one with whom to share his feelings, he is at risk of sinking deep into self-critical thought and depression.

In the worst-case scenario, superempaths reach Harris's fourth life position, 'I'm not OK, you're not OK', a state where they trust no one, not even themselves, which can arise when they have been abused by other people (Harris 1967). Empaths of the highest order are at particular risk of exposure to the threat of abuse by antisocial types. In Chapter 3 we discussed the issue of sociopathic abuse and introduced the idea that sociopathic abuse usually involves three types of people. We called this trio the Sociopath–Empath–Apath Triad (SEAT). Sociopaths often involve empaths in their aggressive dealings because empaths are often highly perceptive. They tend to be hypervigilant to danger and respond to the intimidations of antisocial types and bullies, not on account of their own safety but because of a threat to someone else. This anger, called empathic anger, which we introduced in the last chapter, is a form of empathic distress and is usually felt in a situation where someone else is being hurt by another person or risky circumstance. The sociopathic transaction, which we also discussed in Chapter 3 (pp. 29–32), usually goes something like this: an empath, who sees the situation for what it is, makes a stand on seeing the sociopath say or do something untoward or on perceiving a threatening situation. The empath challenges the sociopath, who tries to throw other people (apaths) off-scent by shifting the blame or focus on to the empath. Thereafter the empath becomes an object of abuse. This scenario and others like it leave the empath feeling at fault, and most likely to consider what he or she might have done wrong before correctly judging the situation.

Living in a world of hostile competitors and apaths leaves the empaths and superempaths among us feeling wounded and somehow defective. Yet how wrong this perspective is! We can all learn from these gifted individuals and their way of being. In the next chapter we consider how to assist superempaths cope better in a hostile world, and we ask them not to lose heart. Many of their everyday relational problems will dissipate when the rest of us finally catch up with them.

10

Helping and valuing the super empathic

Does your daughter get easily overcome watching something sad on television? Does your partner, like Barry, put himself out for others all the time for little to no reward, or often give hard-earned money away to 'good causes' and end up out of pocket? Here we discuss the ups and the downs of being a superempath or living with one in the family. We hope to help you better understand these gifted people, their often extreme reactions to other people and their particular needs with regard to interaction. Superempaths are often easily distracted by the lives and experiences of others – so much so that their reaction can develop as a problem that severely disrupts their lives. Communication with other people can led to stress, anxiety, social phobia, even depression. We include practical strategies to help lessen high empaths' load, heal their wounds and encourage more constructive social interaction.

Giving their power away

Individuals of highly empathic temperament are often kindly and caring. They have a tendency to put others before themselves and it is this that poses the greatest problem. As we highlighted in the previous chapter, empaths, especially extreme ones, can easily find themselves in a position of viewing everyone but themselves as 'OK'. This situation comes about because of their particular attitudes and behaviours. Jack Rosenfeld, author of *Powertake*, sums these tendencies up as an inclination to read too much significance into others' words, a tendency to be non-assertive and a leaning towards fear-driven thinking.

Inclined to read too much into others' words

Highly empathic people are often very sensitive to others' remarks and actions. They tend to try to 'mind read' or second guess others' motives, putting themselves at risk of misinterpreting or reading too much into their words and actions. In addition they may take others' words in ways that aren't meant, or find themselves wounded by the slightest of remarks. This situation can leave a highly empathic person feeling different, vulnerable and flawed.

Highly empathic individuals are often extremely perceptive and intuitive. Most of us are born with some intuitive abilities, and many of us have experienced that sinking feeling when we sense something is wrong – that we or someone we care about is in danger. However, we experience intuition and empathy in varying degrees. What distinguishes the highly attuned is that their empathy button seems stuck on the maximum position – point six – on the empathy spectrum that we discussed in Chapter 2. They experience this ability to tune in as an emotional onslaught that leaves them constantly overwhelmed.

Developing strategies for handling emotionally charged thoughts is important in terms of getting back a sense of control. This is because a surfeit of emotion reeling in the mind can distort an individual's thinking. An example is a work situation where your boss gives you an appraisal and you are told how well you are doing, but you are also told where you could make improvement. Empathic individuals tend to hear only the critical feedback not the praise. They may feel a sense of hurt and view the whole thing as a ticking off or as disapproval.

A tendency to be non-assertive

Empaths can engage in excessive people-pleasing behaviour if they find it too hard to assert their own needs. But a lifelong pattern of people-pleasing can lead to depression and frustration. After all, it can take up a lot of time and energy. Les Carter, in *When Pleasing You is Killing Me*, points out seven distinct signs of people-pleasers that we think apply equally to superempaths.

Have an overdeveloped sense of duty

People-pleasing empaths do what they feel compelled to do or supposed to do, not what they want to do. They give up choice and freedom because they feel obligated to perform certain duties and responsibilities. Living a life of duty is usually unfulfilling – you lose out on experiences and opportunities.

Set aside personal needs

Superempaths too easily set aside the things they need for contentment and success. This can include vital things like money, food, shelter, clothes and emotional needs. People-pleasers discount their own needs, which they view as unimportant. They need to learn that it is OK to say 'No' when someone else's requests interfere with their needs.

Mistake assertiveness for selfishness

Assertiveness is not the same thing as selfishness. Superempaths have often internalized the idea that their decisions may affect the way another person feels, and so avoid being the cause of another person's hurt. Sometimes others are thinking about their priorities, needs and desires. You are responsible for prioritizing yours, not for other people's emotional reactions. People-pleasers often have an overdeveloped conscience and assume too much responsibility for the emotional well-being of others. Learning more self-compassion can restore a balance and help you reach the 'I'm OK, you're OK' status.

Find it difficult to live within limits and boundaries

Everyone is limited to some extent by time, ability, money and other factors, but people-pleasers and superempaths tend to push themselves beyond their limits to keep others happy. Living this way can result in stress, frustration, anger and even financial difficulties. It's important to accept that there are limitations to your resources and generosity. If you don't, you may one day find out the hard way.

Are oversensitive to judgement and criticism

It is a normal, everyday occurrence to be judged by our achievements, beliefs, looks, tastes, social skills, failures and myriad other criteria. Judgements can offer you a gauge of how you are perceived but can be harmful if what others think becomes your measuring stick for your success or failure. Allowing others' views and judgements to take precedence over anything else can lead to anger at yourself and frustration that you fail to live up to their expectations.

Feel the need to control life

Though not all superempaths are easily manipulated, many are. This means they make easy prey for antisocialites like the sociopathic Jill mentioned in Chapters 3 and 4. Some people-pleasers feel the need to be in control, which in times of stress can lead to compulsive behaviours more commonly observed in those of low empathy. Obsessive behaviours and overworking can signify that individuals are trying to empower themselves, particularly if they fear they have lost control of themselves to anxiety and stress. Obsessive and controlling behaviour quickly wears you out.

Aren't honest with themselves

Superempaths never want to be thought of as dishonest, but living to others' expectations and perceptions is a form of deception and allows others to define you and to perpetuate their beliefs about who you are. The dishonest persona serves to distance them emotionally from others because no one really knows who they are. Superempaths are often not true to themselves and can be social chameleons and thus not so far removed from the social dishonest behaviours exhibited by people at the other end of the empathy spectrum – the sociopaths, for example. In order to stop this chameleon-like behaviour it is important to recognize when you are engaging in it. You don't have to become selfish or self-centred – all that is required is for you to cease marching to the beat of someone else's drum and learn to act and behave in ways that suit you best.

Sometimes superempaths go in the opposite direction from non-assertiveness and behave rebelliously in response to feeling wounded. Rebellion can be an open defiance, a passive resistance or an unwillingness to submit to authority. The process often involves feelings of shame and fear, and is a means of trying to reinstate control. It goes something like this: superempaths want people to know they are different from everyone else and are openly defiant; then fear kicks in. Fearing someone may find out how pathetic or unlovable they are, they determine that they must have control of their environment and everyone in it. This is why they try to assert control over their surroundings and other people. If control is threatened in any way, agitation forces them to rebel as a means to regain control. If all attempts at regaining control fail then they may withdraw so that their shame is not exposed and to avoid being controlled.

In the extreme the superempath may reject others entirely and become reclusive, as in the Selfish Giant tale in the last chapter. You might have a family member who behaves like this, such as George, the difficult grandparent we encountered in Chapter 1. Perhaps they stay indoors a lot of the time and you rarely see them out and about. They most likely decline invitations to social events and tend to hide behind closed doors and quietly keep to themselves.

While some time alone is good for everyone, too much can indicate a problem. Where it becomes problematic is where someone becomes a recluse to escape attention or judgement. People like this may stop looking after themselves properly. They may develop unhealthy eating or drinking habits, ignore health concerns and become depressed. Without friends or family to encourage them to find solutions, they may leave troublesome issues unattended until they develop into serious problems. Research indicates that social isolation disrupts people's perceptions about life and affects how they behave and their well-being. Physical health issues that can result from reclusiveness include high blood pressure, increased stress levels, weakened immune system, insomnia, food cravings and drug and alcohol problems.

A propensity for fear-driven thinking

The highly empathic can experience thought as sensation and emotion overload. This can lead to distorted thinking based on fear, worries and insecurities and can affect the way they relate to other people. If this is how you experience everyday life it means you are likely to personalize – take things others say as a criticism of your own character – everyday interactions and experiences. For the highly empathic, learning how to differentiate between random fear and real danger is of great importance. Superempaths may need to learn ways to regulate and manage their 'danger detection' antennae. They must also learn not to internalize everything going on in the outside world, otherwise they risk hiding away captive in their own fortress.

Regaining the balance of power

Some superempaths find themselves in a constant state of anxious excitement, caused by nervous-system arousal. This can lead them to assume they are faulty and malfunctioning and in need of medical help. Indeed, some may be diagnosed with an anxiety disorder – social anxiety, for example, is considered a mental/emotional disorder and some doctors do treat it. Typically this sort of anxiety results from emotional trauma or an ongoing condition that makes social situations particularly difficult. Superempaths tend to be introspective and more attuned to social stimuli, and thus more likely to encounter situations that may lead to their developing social anxiety. But – and this is important – although a superempath can have social anxiety, it doesn't follow that having social anxiety means you're a superempath.

The trouble for the superempath about the medical route is that often intervention starts and ends with anti-anxiety medication. While medicines may seem the simplest and quickest way to see improvements in your well-being, the effects of anti-anxiety medication are usually short-lived. Any drugs that move us under or over our usual state of mental stimulation are likely to be addictive to some degree because they help us get where we want to be with apparent ease. The motives for seeking and using medication are often the same as for drinking too much alcohol, taking non-prescribed and illicit drugs and over- and undereating. All these behaviours are attempts at changing, hopefully for the better, our state of being. The only problem is that none are effective in helping us achieve a healthy state of mind in a lasting way.

For mild to moderate anxiety and depression, the best approach is probably one that combines talking therapies and self-help. In addition, exercise has been proven to help depression, and is one of the main treatments if you have mild depression – your GP may refer you to a qualified fitness trainer for an exercise scheme. Talking through your feelings can be beneficial – it can be either to a friend or relative, or you can ask your GP to suggest a local self-help group. Your GP may also recommend self-help books and online cognitive behavioural therapy (CBT). For more severe depression, medication may be considered in conjunction with talking therapy.

However, if you do consider yourself anxious all the time or in constant low mood, you may be clinically depressed. Depression is more than simply feeling unhappy or fed up – when you're depressed you feel sad for weeks or months rather than just a few days. Depression is an illness with real symptoms. It is not something you can snap out of by pulling yourself together. Nevertheless, with the right treatment and support most people can make a full recovery. The symptoms of depression can be complex and vary widely between people, but they include:

- Continuous low mood or sadness;
- Feeling hopeless and helpless;
- Having low self-esteem;
- Feeling tearful;
- Feeling guilt-ridden;
- Feeling irritable and intolerant of others;
- Having no motivation or interest in things;
- Finding it difficult to make decisions;
- Not getting any enjoyment out of life;
- Feeling anxious or worried;
- Having suicidal thoughts or thoughts of harming yourself.

In addition there may be accompanying physical symptoms, including moving or speaking more slowly than usual and changes in appetite or weight (usually decreased, but sometimes increased), unexplained aches and pains, lack of energy or lack of interest in sex (loss of libido) and disturbed sleep (for example, finding it hard to fall asleep or waking up very early). Socially, people may not do as well at work, take part in fewer social activities, avoid contact with friends and neglect hobbies and interests. They may also experience difficulties in their home and family life.

Things you can do to thrive instead of sinking into depression include reframing your thinking: learning to turn negative and irrational thoughts into more positive ones; learning to stop people-pleasing or avoiding others; developing skills of assertion; and – probably the most important move a superempath can make – learning to be more self-compassionate. These attributes and skills are considered next.

Reframing your thinking

If you have managed to avoid depression but nevertheless suffer with constant anxious thoughts, the good news is that you don't have to accept this as a permanent feature of your makeup. The answer lies in managing the problem from within. You need to develop ways of getting to grips with the emotional turbulence inside and learn how to turn irrational thoughts into rational ones.

The first thing is to tell yourself that you're not defective. The second is to accept your imperfections. You live in a world that doesn't always fully appreciate your gifts of perception and empathy, but there are ways to cope better in an imperfect world. Here are suggestions and advice that others have found useful.

Turning irrational thoughts into rational ones

Examine your fears. You might be afraid that no one will like you, that someone will leave you or that you will be left all alone if you don't say the right thing. If your thoughts have you prisoner, it's time to break out!

A useful method for dealing with the kind of irrational thoughts that refuse to budge is to:

- Pick one of your stubborn irrational thoughts and write it down.
- List anything that suggests the idea is mistaken or false.
- List anything that suggests the idea is true.

In doing this exercise you learn to analyse your irrational thoughts. Afterwards you learn to substitute more **rational self-talk**. Rational self-talk involves more constructive, more realistic and less disapproving thoughts and ideas about yourself and what you can achieve and make possible in everyday life.

Other steps to enable you to reach the optimum 'I'm OK, you're OK' position (see Table 3) include: learning to stop people-pleasing and finding the strength to say 'No' sometimes; learning and putting to the test assertiveness skills; practising more self-compassion.

Table 3 I'm OK, you're OK

I'm OK, you're OK
Belief
I believe and act as if we both deserve respect. We're equally entitled to have things done our way.

Putting a halt to people-pleasing behaviour

By focusing on pleasing others you open yourself up to manipulation and abuse. Conversely, superempaths tend to behave this way to stay safe in their world. If you think you know what those around you are feeling then you know how to adjust what you say and do to make them comfortable so that they are safer people to be around. Superempaths can become social chameleons, shifting conversation styles, choice of tactics and actions to help the people around them feel more at ease. The problem with this is that they often lose track of what are actually their authentic selves. You will never reach your potential as an individual if you constantly hide behind others' expectations, and others will not recognize you for your true worth.

Notice what you're feeling

People-pleasers have often learnt not to consider their feelings, to the extent that they lose touch with them. So the first step in addressing people-pleasing behaviour is to notice what you are feeling.

Assess your boundaries

What is acceptable behaviour for you and what is unacceptable? Do you tolerate the intolerable? Accept the unacceptable? Learn how to identify unacceptable treatment from others and how to set limits on their behaviour when they overstep your boundaries.

Affirm your worth

The person you will spend most time with in this lifetime is yourself, so make the relationship with yourself a positive one. Stop basing your self-worth on how much you do for other people. It's good that you want to help others but it's something you should do because you want to, not because you feel you have to. The willingness to help others should come after you know how to help yourself.

Express your preferences

If you feel that you do so much for others but that they don't do anything for you, maybe it's because you don't express your needs or desires. There's nothing wrong with voicing your opinion or for asking what you want or need. No one can read your mind so it's not fair to make people prise an answer from you. If they ask you what you want, express your preference.

Whenever there is a conflict of desires, try to find a solution that will meet both your needs halfway, or see if there is a win–win situation where both of you can get more than you bargained for.

Learn to say 'No'

Start by finding something not too significant to say 'No' to, and say it firmly. Say it politely, but mean it. You'll be surprised – people rarely take offence. It is best to develop good self-care skills that include healthy assertiveness. You can listen to others, but ultimately what you do is your choice. Keep a balance!

Act on your intuition (gut feelings)

Respect your gut feelings – they're there to help you. Be responsive to them and don't block the messages from within – they are there to alert you to danger or compromising situations.

Practise more self-compassion

Superempaths often are hypercritical of themselves, sometimes because of a lack of self-esteem. If this is you, it might be beneficial to try the following exercise.

Self-compassion exercise 1

Imagine someone who is accepting, kind and compassionate. Imagine that this person can see all your strengths and weaknesses. This person knows all the things that have happened in your life but recognizes the limits of human nature, and is forgiving towards you.

Write a letter to yourself from the perspective of this imaginary person – focusing on the perceived inadequacy for which you tend to judge yourself.

Self-compassion exercise 2

Think about a trait you often criticize yourself for, such as being overly sensitive or anxious or too easily moved to anger. Next answer the following questions:

1 How often do you show this trait? If you don't show it, are you still you?
2 Do certain circumstances bring it out? What are they?
3 Do you have a choice in showing this trait?
4 If you choose not to show it sometimes, how will you behave instead?

What if you were to reframe your description of yourself? For example, you could reframe 'I am an anxious person' to 'Sometimes, in certain circumstances, I get anxious, but at other times I really don't. And in the circumstances when I do get anxious, I can always work on and reduce my irrational thoughts that make me react like that.'

Superempaths and relationships

Superempaths can make great grandparents, partners and siblings. They bring benefits to their intimate relationships, including understanding of their partner's reactions and behaviours. You and your partner will probably feel close to each other (emotional intimacy), and superempaths are capable of creating an environment of trust and safety so vital to intimate and close relationships. However, there is an interesting paradox where superempaths are concerned. Though they might be the most tuned into other people and often the most caring, they are probably the most in need of time away from the rest of us! Judith Orloff, the author of *Emotional Freedom*, describes the highly empathic as a species unto themselves because they absorb their partner's energy and become anxious or exhausted when they don't have time to themselves. Orloff suggests that the highly empathic unwittingly avoid romantic partnership because deep down they're afraid of getting overwhelmed. They want companionship but relationships don't feel particularly safe. However, once they learn to set boundaries and express their preferences, intimacy and deep connections become possible.

For superempaths to be at ease in a relationship they need to assert their needs and indicate what personal space they need in order to thrive. All of us have an invisible boundary that sets a comfort level. If you are a superempath and starting out in a relationship, knowing and communicating what personal boundaries work best for you will stop you from being worn out emotionally by other people. Prospective partners or family members need to know how best to get along with you. You may need to educate them and make things clear. Tell them that this isn't about not loving them – it's about building positive and sustainable relationships. If you're a superempath embarking on a new relationship or trying to re-establish control in an existing one, you might want to take heed of the following tips.

Stand up to people who call you oversensitive

As you're getting to know someone, share with her or him that you're a perceptive person who picks up on things and needs some quiet time once in a while. Don't let others put you down by calling you oversensitive. Yours is a gift, not a fault, so learn to appreciate and value it.

Have at least one quiet room or area in your home in which to retreat

Maintaining your well-being if you're an empath can be challenging if you live with someone else or in a large family. It is a challenge that requires that everyone involved clearly understands the boundaries. Even when extroverts in nature, superempaths tend to need a lot of time alone.

Be unafraid of taking risks and living out of the common way

Superempaths tend to be cooperative rather than competitive, and often underperform in competitive environments. Be prepared to think outside of the box. Although some social interaction is important, superempaths can be effective working unsupervised and make exceptional homeworkers. The same applies to highly empathic children, who may not thrive so well at school but excel if they are educated in the quieter environment of the home, which offers less emotional noise and distraction.

Give yourself time to get things done

Superempaths are easily shaken up and distressed by changes and so need time to adapt to new challenges and situations. Letting go of perfectionism is important – accepting our own imperfections and limitations sometimes can vastly reduce stress.

Keep an eye on your emotional well-being

Avoid emotional exhaustion by keeping a check on your emotional and physical well-being. Problems and anxiety can become magnified when you are fatigued and tired, so getting plenty of physical exercise and a good night's sleep can make a real difference in conquering those worries, and should help you manage your anxiety better.

Keeping hold of a sense of fun

Having the whole world on one's shoulders doesn't tend to make for a whole lot of fun. Letting your hair down and recapturing a sense of fun should help you keep a sense of perspective. Numerous studies support the view that humour and laughter are therapeutic for relieving tension and anxiety. Humour also appears to buffer an individual against the negative effects of stress.

Superempaths who have learnt to keep in reserve sufficient self-compassion are a wondrous sight to behold, for they are all about the gift of empathy and not self-sacrifice or self-denial. In the next chapter we discuss how empathy is the lifeblood of everyday interaction and breathes new life, love and compassion back into families and improves the quality of family life.

11

Handling your emotional abilities

Although we often hear that opposites attract, a study published in the journal *Evolutionary Psychology* of 760 members of an online dating site showed that most had a preference for a partner with the same sort of personality. This might be true of intimate relations, but we don't choose our families. There are always going to be some people in the family with whom we struggle, and others we find easy company.

Whether we are forging new relationships or struggling with old ones and family, it's important to take heed of our inner dialogue and listen to our gut feelings about our relationships. Nothing is going to help you as much as being guided by your own thoughts and feelings. Some types of relationship work well together and some are ill-advised. In the table overleaf we highlight particularly unhealthy matches – we call these by the French term **liaisons dangereuses** (dangerous liaisons). Next to these we highlight more promising matches that have the potential to be wholesome, where both parties have the chance of flourishing. We call these more promising matches **bons amis**, 'good friends' (see Table 4).

In *Les Liaisons dangereuses* by Pierre Choderlos de Laclos, the central character is the Marquise de Merteuil, who seems virtuous and upstanding but is in fact an amoral schemer with a vast sexual appetite. Her malevolent nature is kept well hidden behind a façade of moral righteousness that deceives almost everyone, although in the end her scheming gets the better of her and she falls from grace. Today we might call her a sociopath, psychopath, narcissist or an antisocialite at point zero on the empathy spectrum.

Bon amis imply relationships and affinities of mutual benefit. There is an emotional connection between the individuals and the relationship has a happy balance. Good friends offer amity and companionship. This is more likely when the individuals concerned have good levels of empathy and rate themselves as valuable individuals as well as capable friends or kin.

Table 4 Liaisons dangereuses and bons amis

Liaisons dangereuses	Bons amis
Antisocialites and empaths	Empaths and low empaths
Antisocialites and antisocialites	Empaths and in-betweeners

Liaisons dangereuses

Antisocialite and empath

High-functioning antisocialites may desire to have a relationship or start a family but may be unable to sustain one. The short-lived nature of their relationships is usually due to their becoming bored or sabotaging the relationship, or to their partner becoming unable to tolerate their behaviour. It is possible for an antisocialite such as a psychopath or sociopath to have a long-term relationship where both parties at least appear relatively happy, but they are the exception rather than the rule.

One enduring relationship between an antisocialite and an empath is that of the self-confessed and convicted corporate criminal, psychopath Sam Vaknin, who was the subject of a 2009 documentary film, *I, Psychopath*, which documents his being tested to see if he was born without a conscience. He says he can't empathize with others and is pompous, contradictory and devoid of scruples. He is confirmed by the world's leading experts on psychopathy to be a genuine psychopath. Accompanying Vaknin on the quest for a diagnosis is his long-suffering wife, Lidija. She, like Vaknin, is subjected to a battery of tests, but hers show that she is highly empathic, highly emotional and generous – in other words, an empath.

What is surprising is that when asked about her perception of her husband, Lidija asserts that he is not abusive. Vaknin's view of his wife and their marriage, on the other hand, is clinical and cold. He asserts that he is incapable of loving her and despite her wish for a baby he insists they will never have a child. He practically scoffs at her for her loyalty and for staying in what he regards as a one-sided relationship. To the outsider looking in, and despite her insistence that theirs is a good marriage, she appears to be completely in thrall to her husband. This is not a vision of a happy and loving union but it does probably reflect something of Lidija's take on life. She comes across as world-weary and more than a little resigned to a life of unrequited love.

While empaths and antisocialites are not usually a good mix, there is possibly one exception. In cases where one person has borderline personality disorder (BPD) or some mild antisocial traits but is capable of love and affection, positive relations can be forged as long as effective boundaries are in place. This means that both parties need to be clear about the rules of engagement. Empaths need to balance between empathy and independence – to resolve not to end up as scapegoats while living with someone who idealizes them one minute and devalues and criticizes them the next. Research shows that people with BPD and other conditions of emotional instability tend to have stormy romantic and platonic relations, but as long as everyone understands what to expect, it is possible to share healthy relationships. The key is to be open about the problems that can result from the dichotomous – black and white – thinking, to encourage the person with emotional instability to get professional help.

Antisocialite and antisocialite

Another liaison dangereuse to avoid at all costs is that between one antisocialite and another – for example, between someone who has a hefty dose of narcissism and another with traits of BPD or emotional instability. Such people may feel naturally drawn to someone with whom they have an outlook in common or who echoes personality aspects in themselves. Narcissistic personality types can confuse others with their overly generous ways, which seem out of keeping with their selfishness and lack of personal boundaries. In relationships, or as parents, they often avoid intimacy and closeness. Individuals with BPD and narcissistic types in close proximity are highly likely to trample on each other's emotions and trigger highly explosive episodes, while remaining hopelessly enmeshed.

Another antisocialite–antisocialite combination that is dangerous is sociopaths intermixing with sociopaths. Sociopaths tend to interact with other sociopaths in a predatory way and in competition with other antisocialites. They are rarely attracted to one another for the sake of positive relations, and feel no reason to interact unless they have a common goal or can benefit from mutual collaboration. One such situation is when they have their sights set on the same target. This situation can occur in families where more than one member of the group is sociopathic or narcissistic. In such situations the bullies within the family, especially female bullies, tend to manipulate people through their emotions – such as guilt – and through their beliefs, attitudes and perceptions, and see any form of vulnerability as an opportunity for manipulation. Those especially prone to exploitation under such circumstances include empaths and the highly perceptive (because they pose a threat to the sociopath's dominance); however, elderly relatives, the young and those with infirmity or illness also are potential targets.

Bons amis

Empaths and low empaths can often forge healthy and lasting relationships. Empaths who have good listening skills, patience and compassion are often invaluable support to low empaths, and can be especially helpful to those with restricted social skills – for example, a partner with Asperger syndrome, which we discussed in Chapters 2 and 5. A relative or partner who is willing to explain things, sometimes over and over again, and not criticize, can help enormously as the other person attempts to build confidence and social skills. Conversely empaths, especially the superempathic kind, can benefit from the kind of down-to-earth, no-nonsense approach of the low empath, and being around people who aren't afraid of standing apart or being assertive and saying 'No'.

Superempaths and in-betweeners – those with low to middling empathy – can also help each other out. For example, a superempath may learn from an in-betweener to respond less emotionally to a situation, or the in-betweener may learn compassion or empathic outrage from a superempath.

Building a culture of empathy and cooperation

Self-absorption in all its forms kills empathy, let alone compassion. When we focus on ourselves, our world contracts as our problems and preoccupations loom large. But when we focus on others, our world expands. Our own problems drift to the periphery of the mind and so seem smaller, and we increase our capacity for connection – or compassionate action.

So says Daniel Goleman in *Social Intelligence: The New Science of Human Relationships* (2006). Whether we are aware of it or not, many of us are ensconced in a culture of blame, where those who don't fit the mould or refuse to fit in are usually ostracized for being different. A blame game ensues, which can be a serious problem for the vulnerable, noncompliant or weak and those who can't defend themselves. Feelings of guilt, aggression, culpability and suffering are transferred from one family member or group to another in an attempt to resolve or avoid bad feelings. It is in this way that responsibility and blame are displaced.

In general people behave badly towards one another because they can't feel what they are doing to others. In effect their sense of 'other' is missing. This lack of sensitivity is not in itself sufficient to lead to cruelty, but it is an essential element. To get our sensibilities in order we need to acquire more self-awareness. Self-awareness means having a clear perception of your personality – your thoughts, beliefs, motivation and emotions. Self-awareness allows you to understand yourself and by doing so it is possible to understand other people and your responses to them better. Learning to be more attentive in this way pays dividends because it means you will become more aware of how you are in relation to other people.

Self-awareness needs coupling with self-compassion. Self-compassion is described by the psychologist Kristin Neff as having three elements: self-kindness; common humanity; mindfulness. Self-compassionate people recognize that failure and life difficulties are inevitable, but tend to be gentle with themselves rather than angry when life falls short of the ideal. Suffering and personal failure are viewed as part of our shared human experience, with a balanced approach to our negative emotions so that feelings are neither suppressed nor exaggerated. Research suggests that giving ourselves a break and accepting our imperfections may be the first step towards better health. Self-compassion is a skill we can learn and practise.

Another useful skill is learning to listen actively to and acknowledge others, which increases the chance that others will be willing to listen in turn. Listening is one way of showing ongoing appreciation and encouragement of others and helps build a stronger relationship.

In the end what makes empathy a positive and prosocial phenomenon is that at its core rests human decency and morality. Sometimes we ignore our conscience and feelings of concern for others, but thankfully most of us are unable to silence our empathy for long. Silenced empathy has a deeply disturbing and destabilizing effect on society. Empathy is not something we are born with.

Learning from experience and a desire to connect deeply with other people, we can become skilled at stepping into another person's reality. These skills are part of compassionate communication, the fundamentals of which, thankfully, most of us have. Mindfully employing these skills means we become more competent empaths. Jointly this supports us in building a culture of empathy, one that enables us to achieve and derive mutual benefit.

Encouragingly, a study by a team of researchers at the University of North Carolina suggests that being a good friend, and being compassionate, may be among the best ways to improve your own health. The study suggests that giving and receiving social support translates into physical benefits such as lower blood pressure, healthier weight and other physiological measures of sound health. According to the research, many indirect clues point to relationships being healing. This suggests that every positive interaction we have with people benefits our health (Kok et al. 2013).

Lastly, while research indicates that women tend to exhibit higher levels of empathy than men, this is probably due to differing cultural expectations put upon men and women, rather than any fundamental difference. It is therefore a mistake to assume that males and females have different capacities for empathy. All of us can develop our communication skills, so the message is not to give up. Empathy and helping behaviour increase with age.

12

Families have the final say

Here are some words from families about coping with some fairly difficult behaviour. It's heartening to see how each family has worked out ways of contending with the difficulties facing them, and succeeded in enhancing the quality of family life.

Sally

My sister struggles with her emotions, has mood swings and sometimes threatens to harm herself. She's been doing this since her early teens and is now 19. Often she phones and texts repeatedly when she is upset and feels like hurting herself. I find this deeply distressing and I felt overburdened with her problems. She tests me out all the time, and says unpleasant things to push me away. I know she doesn't really mean it; it's just her way. Recently I read online about borderline personality disorder, which is what is behind the self-harming and other issues she's got, at least that's what I think anyway. I came across the NHS Choices website, which was helpful, and the organization Mind's website. Both websites give lots of useful advice. I've since discussed it with my sister. She was reluctant at first but a few weeks ago she had an appointment with her GP and spoke about the self-harming for the first time to a professional. I realize I have to stop taking on all her problems, which I can't handle anyway. And for her it's about learning to help herself with proper support and counselling.

Gary

When I was young I was one of those sorts who followed the crowd and I ended up in a gang. As I got older I wanted to go my own way, only it was hard at that stage to make a stand. I managed eventually, and this is what I did. The first thing was that I stopped dressing like a member of the gang and then began to isolate myself from the other members. I took public transport instead of walking and avoided places where the gang hung out. I figured it was a case of 'out of sight, out of mind'. I didn't tell anyone from the gang about my plans to leave, and wouldn't advise anyone to tell anyone, ever. Fellow gang members can never be fully trusted. The best thing I did was move away from the area. I never went back again. When I look back I realize I was scared a lot of the time and the fear stopped me doing right by myself. I'm really glad I left the gang in the end. Nowadays I've a good life, a good job and kids of my own. Not so long ago – sometime last year – I helped set up a gang-avoidance project in the local neighbourhood. I talk to kids about not following others, being a bit of a sheep like I was, and instead leading their own lives. I want to instil in my kids more self-respect and confidence so they resist gang-life.

Jenny

Our children say their father is a right old grump and tease him about it. He is obsessional about things and is sensitive to smells and noise. He gets stressed if anyone tries to change things and is really obsessed with routine. Woe betide anyone who tries to change things at home! Sometimes he will say outlandish things but doesn't realize that his remarks are offensive, and he's forever winding people up, especially strangers, though it's usually unintentional.

I've wondered before if he has a mild form of Asperger but he's not keen to discuss it. Anyway, we've learnt to deal with his behaviour in a way that works for us. Sometimes if he oversteps the mark and winds me up I explain why his actions bother me (he doesn't usually get why I'm upset, you see). The children are good with him, and bring humour to the situation. We call him our very own Victor Meldrew – the character from the television series *One Foot in the Grave*. He doesn't mind too much that we take the mickey. We know he doesn't mean to cause offence; it's just he does fixate on things. I'm learning to reframe things. I try not to get upset and angry or view all of his actions negatively. We often have disagreements but we are moving forwards. Nowadays I'm much more specific and direct about what he's done that bothers me. I write him short notes sometimes to spell out what the issue is and what would resolve it. That seems to help. He's not so good at heart to hearts or that sort of thing. One good thing about our relationship is that I'm a very emotional person, too emotional sometimes, so I guess we balance each another out! Our relationship is pretty good these days.

Richard

My mother-in-law is totally selfish and narcissistic! Early on when we first got married my wife used to cave in to her mother's demands and that would cause us to fall out. Once she invited herself on holiday with us! She literally turned up unannounced at our house with her suitcase packed! Nowadays my wife is more willing to say 'No' when her demands are excessive. We've found getting angry with her only makes things worse. What we do now is frame things differently. Instead of saying to her, 'We'd prefer you didn't coming on holiday with us', we reframe it as, 'We'd love it if you would come and stay when we've returned from our holiday.' She might protest and overstep the mark from time to time, but we've learnt that being firm and consistent is what helps makes things more bearable. Keeping our cool and a sense of humour helps – a lot!

Richard and his wife fared better than most by putting in place good boundaries. Laura's mother, from Chapter 1, could be dealt with in much the same way. And perhaps the situation for the family of 80-year-old George, who stopped all contact with his family and then died, might have ended more positively had boundaries been instigated years before.

Liz

Our son is very perceptive and absorbs everything going on around him, including other people's moods. He's friendly – in fact what is so attractive about him is his kind heart and affable nature. As he's got older he prefers to spend a lot of time on his own. He says he needs his space. If he's around people all the time he quite often becomes overwhelmed by their problems. This was a significant problem for him in his early teens – he ended up attracting a lot of needy people. Nowadays he is more assertive and takes more care of himself. This sounds a bit silly really, but to help him along we bought him a mug with the words, 'I love me' written on it. We wanted him to remember to put himself first sometimes! He's doing fine these days. He's got the balance right.

Harry

When Grandma divorced Granddad at the age of 60 she spent the entire divorce settlement on an apartment in Spain. Things changed because we didn't see a lot of her from then on as she left the UK for good. Whenever we tried to arrange a time to chat on Skype she was always too busy to talk for long, and when we asked if we could visit her in Spain her answer was always full of excuses as to why it just wasn't OK. It felt like she was pushing us away. I felt rejected and I guess my brothers did as well. One day, in exasperation, Mum wrote Grandma a letter telling her how much we all missed her. Then Mum flew out to see her in person to explain how we all felt and that we were worried about losing contact. It seemed to do the trick. Nowadays we have a lot more contact. She's even promised to come and visit us soon. It's all good.

It really does seem from these accounts from families with difficult members that empathy and effective boundaries are the keys to constructive relations.

Useful addresses

General

Al-Anon
Helpline: 020 7403 0888 (10 a.m. to 10 p.m., 365 days a year)
Website: www.al-anonuk.org.uk
For families in the UK and Eire affected by someone's drinking. Alateen, part of Al-Anon, is for teenagers who are affected.

Alcoholics Anonymous
Helpline: 0845 769 7555
Website: www.alcoholics-anonymous.org.uk
For families and friends, see also **Al-Anon**.

B-eat
Helplines: 0845 634 1414 (adults); 0845 634 7650 (people under 25)
Website: www.b-eat.co.uk
For people with eating disorders.

British Association of Counselling and Psychotherapy
Tel.: 01455 883300 (general enquiries, open during office hours)
Website: www.bacp.co.uk

ChildLine
Helpline: 0800 1111
Website: www.childline.org.uk
This service is provided by the **NSPCC** (see overleaf).

Drinkline
National helpline: 0800 917 8282

GamCare
Helpline: 0808 8020 133 (free, 8 a.m. to midnight, 7 days a week)
Website: www.gamcare.org.uk
Provides support, information and advice to anyone coping with a gambling problem.

Mind
Infoline: 0300 123 3393
Website: www.mind.org.uk
Provides help and support for anyone with a mental-health concern.

National Autistic Society
Helpline: 0808 800 4104 (10 a.m. to 4 p.m., Monday to Friday except bank holidays)
Website: www.autism.org.uk
For people with autism and Asperger syndrome.

National Health Service (NHS Direct: England and Wales)
Helpline: 111 or 0845 46 47
Website: www.nhsdirect.nhs.uk

National Health Service (NHS 24: Scotland)
Helpline: 08454 242424
Website: www.nhs24.com

NHS Choices
Website: www.nhs.uk/Pages/HomePage.aspx

National Society for the Prevention of Cruelty to Children (NSPCC)
Helpline: 0808 800 5000 (for adults concerned about a child)
Website: www.nspcc.org.uk

Samaritans
Helpline: 08457 90 90 90 (24 hours a day, 365 days a year)
Website: www.samaritans.org

Talk to Frank
Helpline: 0800 77 66 00
Website: www.talktofrank.com
For those concerned about drugs.

Websites and internet resources

Center for Building a Culture of Empathy
Website: http://cultureofempathy.com

Free Mindfulness
Website: www.freemindfulness.org/download
Provides mindfulness meditation exercises that are free to download.

Gamblers Anonymous UK
Website: www.gamblersanonymous.org.uk
A fellowship of people who have joined together to do something about their own gambling problem and to help others to do the same, through local meetings.

GET.gg Self Help and Therapist Resources
Website: www.getselfhelp.co.uk
Focuses on cognitive behaviour therapy.

Good Therapy
Website: www.goodtherapy.org/types-of-therapy.html
Based in the USA, this site helps people to find therapists and encourages the use of ethical therapy.

Men Get Eating Disorders Too (MGEDT)
Website: http://mengetedstoo.co.uk

Mental Health Foundation
Website: www.mentalhealth.org.uk/help-information/podcasts/
mindfulness-10-minute/
The Foundation has produced a ten-minute podcast which consists of a relaxation exercise narrated by an expert in mindfulness, Professor Mark Williams, and features a series of breathing and visualization techniques.

PsychologyTools
Website: www.psychologytools.org/compassion-focused-therapy.html
PsychologyTools develops free materials to download, including resources for compassion focused therapy.

SMART Recovery UK
Website: www.smartrecovery.org.uk
For people recovering from addictive behaviour.

References

Aron, E. N., *The Highly Sensitive Person: How to Thrive When the World Overwhelms You* (New York: Carol Publishing, 1996).

Aron, E. N., Aron, A. and Jagiellowicz, J. (2012), 'Sensory Processing Sensitivity: A Review in the Light of the Evolution of Biological Responsivity', *Personality and Social Psychology Review* 16(3): 262–82.

Attwood, T. et al., *Asperger's and Girls* (Arlington, TX: Future Horizons, 2006).

Cleckley, H. M., *The Mask of Sanity* (St Louis, MO: C. V. Mosby Co., 1941).

Derntl, B., Seidel, E-M., Schneider, F. and Habel, U. (2012), 'How Specific are Emotional Deficits? A Comparison of Empathic Abilities in Schizophrenia, Bipolar and Depressed Patients', *Schizophrenia Research* 142(1–3): 58–64.

De Sousa, A., McDonald, S., Rushby, J., Li, S., Dimoska, A. and James, C. (2011), 'Understanding Deficits in Empathy after Traumatic Brain Injury: The Role of Affective Responsivity', *Cortex* 47(5): 526.

Goleman, D., *Emotional Intelligence* (New York: Bantam Books, 1995).

Goleman, D., *Working with Emotional Intelligence* (New York: Bantam Books, 1998).

Goleman, D., *Social Intelligence: The New Science of Human Relationships* (New York: Bantam Books, 2006).

Hambrook, D., Tchanturia, K., Schmidt, U., Russell, T. and Treasure, J. (2008), 'Empathy, Systemizing, and Autistic Traits in Anorexia Nervosa: A Pilot Study', *British Journal of Clinical Psychology* 47: 335–9. See also Russell, T. A., Schmidt, U., Doherty, L., Young, V., Tchanturia, K. (2009), 'Aspects of Social Cognition in Anorexia Nervosa: Affective and Cognitive Theory of Mind', *Psychiatry Research* 168(3): 181–5.

Harris, Thomas A., *I'm OK – You're OK* (London: Arrow Books, 2012; first published New York: Harper & Row, 1967).

Kagan, J., *Galen's Prophecy: Temperament in Human Nature* (New York: Basic Books, 1998).

Kok, B. E., Coffey, K. A., Cohn, M. A., Catalino, L. I., Vacharkulksemsuk, T., Algoe, S. B., Brantley, M. and Fredrickson, B. L. (2013), 'How Positive Emotions Build Physical Health: Perceived Positive Social Connections Account for the Upward Spiral Between Positive Emotions and Vagal Tone', *Psychological Science* 24(7): 1123–32.

Mayer, J. D. and Stevens, A. A. (1994), 'An Emerging Understanding of the Reflective (Meta-) Experience of Mood', *Journal of Research in Personality* 28(3): 351–73.

Moehler, E., Kagan, J., Oelkers-Ax, R., Brunner, R., Poustka, L., Haffner, J. and Resch, F. (2008), 'Infant Predictors of Behavioral Inhibition', *British Journal of Developmental Psychology* 26(1): 145–50.

Rogers, K., Dziobek, I., Hassenstab, J., Wolf, O. T. and Convit, J. A. (2007),

'Who Cares? Revisiting Empathy in Asperger Syndrome', *Journal of Autism and Developmental Disorders* 37: 709–15.

Sack, D., 'What Makes Addicts Stop Caring? How Empathy gets Hijacked by Addiction' (14 Nov. 2011), <www.selfgrowth.com/articles/what-makes-addicts-stop-caring-how-empathy-gets-hijacked-by-addiction>

Savage, E., *Don't Take It Personally! The Art of Dealing with Rejection* (Lincoln, NE: iUniverse, 2002; first published Oakland, CA: New Harbinger Publications, 1997).

Smoller, J. W., Craddock, N., Kendler, K., Lee, P. H., Neale, B. M., Nurnberger, J. I., Ripke, S., Santangelo, S. and Sullivan, P. F. (2013), 'Identification of Risk Loci with Shared Effects on Five Major Psychiatric Disorders: A Genome-wide Analysis', *Lancet* 381(9875): 1371–9.

Further reading

Attwood, T., *The Complete Guide to Asperger Syndrome* (London: Jessica Kingsley, 2008).

Babiak, P. and Hare, R. D., *Snakes in Suits* (New York: Collins, 2006).

Baron-Cohen, S., *Zero Degrees of Empathy: A New Theory of Human Cruelty* (London: Allen Lane, 2011).

Behary, W. T., *Disarming the Narcissist: Surviving and Thriving with the Self-Absorbed* (Oakland CA: New Harbinger, 2008).

Boyd, B., *Appreciating Asperger Syndrome: Looking at the Upside – With 300 Positive Points* (London: Jessica Kingsley, 2009).

Brown, B., *The Gifts of Imperfection: Let Go of Who You Think You're Supposed to Be and Embrace Who You Are* (Minnesota: Hazelden, 2010).

Carter, L., *When Pleasing You is Killing Me: A Workbook* (Nashville, TN: B & H Publishing Group, 2007).

Chapman, A. L. and Gratz, K. L., *The Borderline Personality Disorder Survival Guide: Everything You Need to Know About Living with BPD* (Oakland, CA: New Harbinger, 2007).

Davis, L., *I thought We'd Never Speak Again: The Road from Estrangement to Reconciliation* (New York: HarperCollins, 2002).

Fjelstad, M., *Stop Caretaking the Borderline or Narcissist: How to End the Drama and Get on with Life* (Lanham, MD; Plymouth: Rowman & Littlefield, 2013).

Forward, S. and Buck, S., *Toxic Parents: Overcoming Their Hurtful Legacy and Reclaiming Your Life* (New York: Bantam Books, 2002).

Goleman, D., *Emotional Intelligence* and *Working with Emotional Intelligence*, omnibus edn (London: Bloomsbury Publishing, 2004).

Jolin, L., *Coping with Drug Problems in the Family* (London: Sheldon Press, 2012).

Keysers, C., *The Empathic Brain* (Netherlands: Social Brain Press, 2011).

Kreisman, J. J. and Straus, H., *I Hate You – Don't Leave Me* (New York: HarperCollins, 1991).

Krznaric, R., *The Wonderbox: Curious Histories of How to Live* (London: Profile Books, 2011).

Lerner, R., *The Object of My Affection is in My Reflection: Narcissists and Their Relationships* (Florida: Health Communications, 2009).

McGregor, J. and McGregor, T., *The Empathy Trap: Understanding Antisocial Personalities* (London: Sheldon Press, 2013).

Marshall, F., *Living with Autism* (London: Sheldon Press, 2004).

Mason, P. T. and Kreger, R., *Stop Walking on Eggshells: Taking Your Life Back When Someone You Care About Has Borderline Personality Disorder* (Oakland CA: New Harbinger, 2010).

Neff, K., *Self-compassion: Stop Beating Yourself up and Leave Insecurity Behind* (NY: HarperCollins, 2011).

Nowak, M. and Highfield, R., *Supercooperators: Beyond the Survival of the Fittest: Why Cooperation, Not Competition, is the Key to Life* (Edinburgh: Canongate Books, 2011).

Orloff, J., *Emotional Freedom: Liberate Yourself from Negative Emotions and Transform Your Life* (New York: Three Rivers Press, 2011).

Ramachandran, V., *The Tell-tale Brain Unlocking the Mystery of Human Nature: Tales of the Unexpected from Inside Your Mind* (London: Heinemann, 2011).

Rosenfeld, J., *Powertake: Get What You Want Without Hurting Others* (New York: Universe, 2010).

Roth, K. and Freidman, F. B., *Surviving a Borderline Parent: How to Heal Your Childhood Wounds and Build Trust, Boundaries and Self-esteem* (Oakland CA: New Harbinger, 2003).

Searle, R., *Asperger Syndrome in Adults: A Guide to Realizing your Potential* (London: Sheldon Press, 2010).

Stern, R., *The Gaslight Effect: How to Spot and Survive the Hidden Manipulation Others Use to Control your Life* (New York: Morgan Road Books, 2007).

Stout, M., *The Sociopath Next Door* (New York: Broadway Books, 2005).

Index